Dementia

A Comprehensive Guide to Understanding, Diagnosis, and Treatment

Ethan D. Anderson

Xspurts.com

A New Zealand Designed Product

Other Versions Available

Why limit yourself to just one format?

This book is now available in physical, digital, and audiobook options.

Choose the way you love to read and dive into the story today. You won't regret it!

Digital ISBN: 9781776969272
Physical ISBN: 9781776969265
Audio ISBN:

To obtain a different format of this book at a discounted price, please get in touch with us at:

http://isbn.xspurts.com/

Contents

Have Questions / Comments?

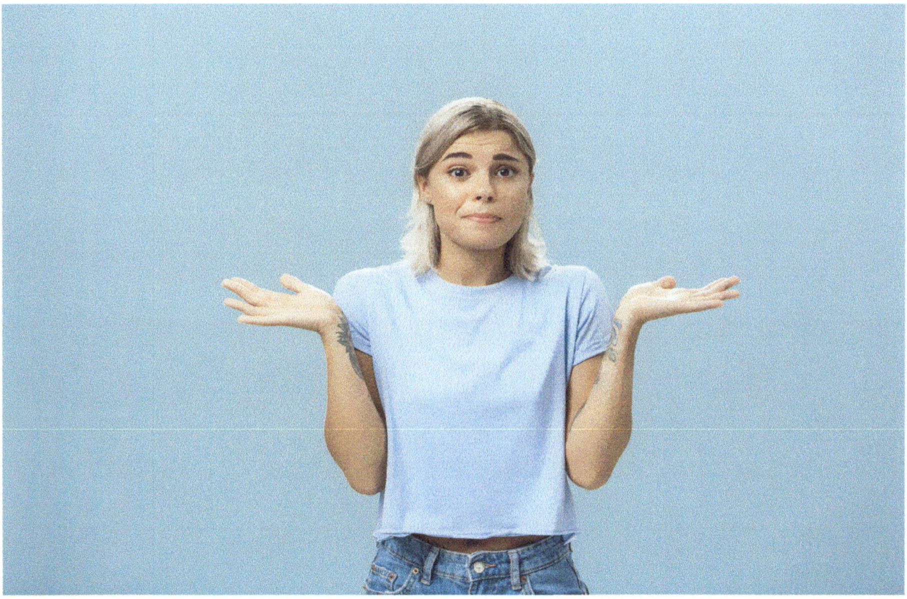

This book was designed to cover as much information as possible, but I know I have probably missed something, or some new amazing discovery has just come out.

If you notice something missing or have a question that I failed to answer, please get in touch and let me know. If I can, I will email you an answer and also update the book so others can also benefit from it.

Thanks For Being Awesome :)

Submit Your Questions / Comments At:

https://questions.xspurts.com

Get Free Stuff

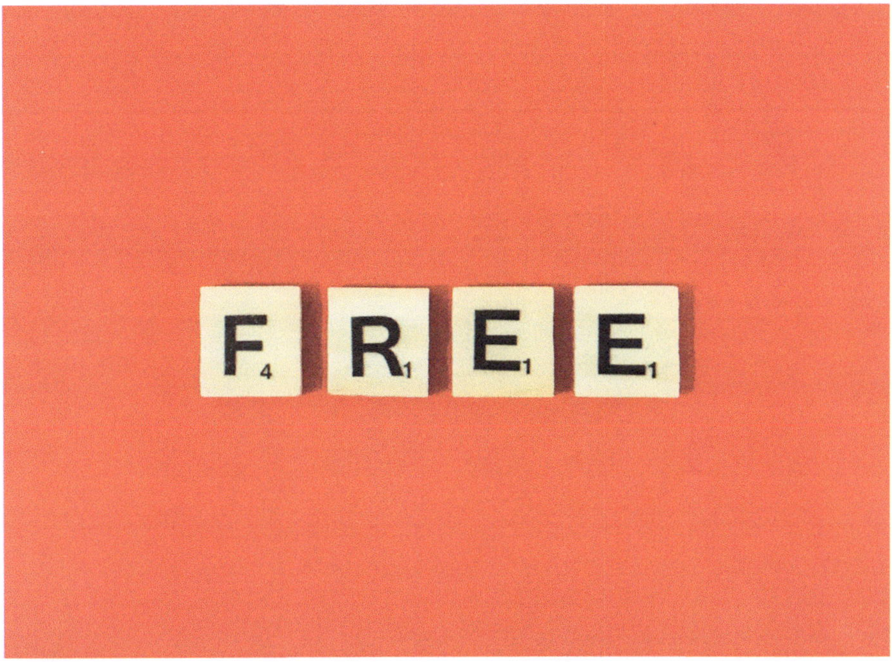

We love writing and have produced a huge number of books.

For being one of our amazing readers, we would love to offer you more books we have created, 100% free.

To claim this limited time special offer, simply go to the site below and enter your name and email address.

You will then receive loads (as we love our readers so much :) of our great books, content and audio direct to your email account, 100% free!

Get Loads of FREE Stuff at:

https://free.xspurts.com

Chapter One

Understanding Dementia

Dementia is a broad term used to describe a range of cognitive impairments that affect memory, thinking, behavior, and emotions. It is a progressive and degenerative condition that affects people's ability to perform daily activities, and it is estimated to affect more than 50 million people worldwide. While dementia is most commonly associated with aging, it is not a normal part of the aging process. Below we will we will explore what dementia is, its causes, symptoms, and available treatments.

Dementia is caused by damage to the brain cells, which interferes with the normal functioning of the brain. This damage can be caused by a variety of factors, including genetics, age, lifestyle, and environmental factors. Alzheimer's disease is the most common cause of dementia, accounting for up to 70% of cases. Other causes include vascular dementia, Lewy body dementia, frontotemporal dementia, and Parkinson's disease.

The symptoms of dementia can vary depending on the cause and stage of the disease, but generally include memory loss, difficulty communicating, confusion, mood changes, and difficulty performing daily activities. In the early stages of the disease, symptoms may be mild and easily overlooked, but as the disease progresses, they become more severe and noticeable.

One of the challenges of diagnosing dementia is that many of the symptoms overlap with other conditions, such as depression or medication side effects. To make a diagnosis, doctors will conduct a variety of tests, including neurological and cognitive exams, blood tests, and brain imaging scans. Early diagnosis is important because it allows for early treatment and management of the disease.

Currently, there is no cure for dementia, but there are treatments available that can help manage symptoms and slow the progression of the disease. Medications such as cholinesterase inhibitors and memantine are commonly prescribed to help with memory and cognitive function. Lifestyle changes such as exercise, a healthy diet, and social activities can also help improve symptoms and quality of life for people with dementia.

In addition to medication and lifestyle changes, there are also non-pharmacological interventions that can be helpful for people with dementia. Cognitive stimulation therapy, reminiscence therapy, and music therapy have all been shown to improve cognitive function and quality of life for people with dementia.

Caring for someone with dementia can be challenging and stressful, but there are resources and support available for caregivers. Support groups, respite care, and professional caregiving services can all provide assistance and relief for caregivers.

One of the best ways to prevent or delay the onset of dementia is to maintain a healthy lifestyle. Eating a healthy diet, exercising regularly, getting enough sleep, and staying socially active are all important for maintaining brain health. Additionally, avoiding smoking and excessive alcohol consumption can also help reduce the risk of developing dementia.

In conclusion, dementia is a complex and challenging condition that affects millions of people worldwide. While there is currently no cure for the disease, there are treatments available that can help manage symptoms and improve quality of life for people with dementia. Early diagnosis and management of the disease are crucial for ensuring the best possible outcomes for patients and their caregivers. By maintaining a healthy lifestyle and staying socially active, individuals can reduce their risk of developing dementia and improve their overall brain health.

Definition and types of dementia

Dementia is a term used to describe a group of symptoms related to cognitive decline and memory loss. It is not a specific disease, but rather a collection of symptoms caused by a variety of underlying conditions. Dementia affects millions of people worldwide, and its prevalence is expected to increase in the coming years due to the aging of the population. Below we will we will explore the definition and types of dementia.

The term "dementia" refers to a decline in cognitive function and memory that is severe enough to interfere with daily activities. It is not a normal part of aging, but rather a symptom of an underlying disease or condition. While dementia is most commonly associated with memory loss, it can also affect other cognitive functions, such as language, reasoning, and judgment.

There are several types of dementia, each with its own unique set of symptoms and underlying causes. Alzheimer's disease is the most common type of dementia, accounting for up to 70% of cases. It is a progressive and irreversible brain disease that affects memory, thinking, and behavior. The exact cause of Alzheimer's disease is not fully understood, but it is believed to be caused by a combination of genetic, environmental, and lifestyle factors.

Vascular dementia is the second most common type of dementia, accounting for up to 20% of cases. It is caused by a reduction in blood flow to the brain, often due to a stroke or other cardiovascular disease. Symptoms of vascular dementia can include memory loss, difficulty with language and communication, and problems with motor skills.

Lewy body dementia is another type of dementia that is caused by abnormal protein deposits in the brain. It can cause a range of symptoms, including hallucinations, sleep disturbances, and problems with movement and balance. Lewy body dementia is often misdiagnosed as Alzheimer's disease or Parkinson's disease, but it has its own unique set of symptoms and treatment options.

Frontotemporal dementia is a less common type of dementia that affects the frontal and temporal lobes of the brain. It can cause changes in personality and behavior, as well as problems with language and communication. Frontotemporal dementia is often diagnosed at a younger age than other types of dementia, typically in people in their 50s and 60s.

Parkinson's disease is a progressive neurological disorder that can also cause dementia. It is caused by the degeneration of dopamine-producing neurons in the brain, which can lead to tremors, stiffness, and problems with movement. In addition to motor symptoms, Parkinson's disease can also cause cognitive impairment and dementia.

Other less common types of dementia include Huntington's disease, Creutzfeldt-Jakob disease, and Wernicke-Korsakoff syndrome. Each of these types of dementia has its own unique set of symptoms and underlying causes.

In conclusion, dementia is a group of symptoms related to cognitive decline and memory loss that can be caused by a variety of underlying conditions. There are several types of dementia, each with its own unique set of symptoms and causes. Alzheimer's disease is the most common type of dementia, but there are other types, including vascular dementia, Lewy body dementia, frontotemporal dementia, and Parkinson's disease. Early diagnosis and management of the disease are crucial for ensuring the best possible outcomes for patients and their caregivers.

The stages of dementia and progression

Dementia is a progressive and degenerative condition that affects memory, thinking, behavior, and emotions. It is a complex and challenging disease that can be difficult to manage, and it can have a significant impact on the lives of patients and their caregivers. Below we will we will explore the stages of dementia and its progression.

The progression of dementia can vary depending on the type of dementia and the individual patient, but there are generally four stages of dementia that are commonly recognized. These stages are mild cognitive impairment, early-stage dementia, middle-stage dementia, and late-stage dementia.

Mild cognitive impairment is the earliest stage of dementia. At this stage, the patient may experience mild memory loss and cognitive decline, but their symptoms are not severe enough to interfere with daily activities. Mild cognitive impairment is not always a precursor to dementia, but it can be a warning sign.

Early-stage dementia is the second stage of the disease. At this stage, the patient's symptoms become more noticeable and begin to interfere with daily activities. They may experience difficulty with memory, communication, and problem-solving. The patient may also begin to experience mood changes and personality changes.

Middle-stage dementia is the third stage of the disease. At this stage, the patient's symptoms become more severe, and they may require assistance with daily activities. They may experience significant memory loss and confusion, and they may have difficulty communicating. Behavioral symptoms, such as wandering, agitation, and aggression, may also become more common.

Late-stage dementia is the final stage of the disease. At this stage, the patient's symptoms are severe, and they require round-the-clock care. They may no longer be able to communicate verbally and may be confined to a wheelchair or bed. They may also experience difficulty swallowing and have an increased risk of infections and other complications.

The progression of dementia can be influenced by a variety of factors, including the underlying cause of the disease, the age of the patient, and the patient's overall health. Some patients may progress through the stages of dementia more quickly than others, while others may progress more slowly.

In addition to the four stages of dementia, there are also several sub-stages that are used to describe the progression of the disease in more detail. These sub-stages include the preclinical stage, the prodromal stage, and the severe stage. Each of these sub-stages is characterized by different symptoms and levels of severity.

The preclinical stage of dementia is the earliest stage of the disease, and it is characterized by the presence of biomarkers that indicate the development of the disease. At this stage, the patient may not experience any symptoms, but the disease is already affecting the brain.

The prodromal stage of dementia is the stage between mild cognitive impairment and early-stage dementia. At this stage, the patient's symptoms are more noticeable, but they are not severe enough to interfere with daily activities.

The severe stage of dementia is the final stage of the disease, and it is characterized by severe cognitive decline, behavioral symptoms, and a high level of dependence on caregivers. At this stage, the patient requires round-the-clock care and may no longer be able to communicate verbally.

In conclusion, dementia is a progressive and degenerative condition that affects millions of people worldwide. The progression of the disease can vary depending on the type of dementia and the individual patient, but there are generally four stages of dementia that are commonly recognized. These stages include mild cognitive impairment, early-stage dementia, middle-stage dementia, and late-stage dementia. Early diagnosis and management of the disease are crucial for ensuring the best possible outcomes for patients and their caregivers.

Common symptoms and early warning signs

Dementia is a progressive and degenerative condition that affects memory, thinking, behavior, and emotions. It can be a challenging disease to manage, and early diagnosis and management are crucial for ensuring the best possible outcomes for patients and their caregivers. Below we will we will explore the common symptoms and early warning signs of dementia.

One of the earliest signs of dementia is mild cognitive impairment. At this stage, the patient may experience mild memory loss and cognitive decline, but their symptoms are not severe enough to interfere with daily activities. They may have difficulty remembering names, dates, or events, and they may have trouble with problem-solving and decision-making.

As the disease progresses, the patient's symptoms become more noticeable and begin to interfere with daily activities. Early-stage dementia is characterized by significant memory loss and confusion. The patient may have difficulty finding words, following conversations, or completing familiar tasks. They may also experience mood changes, such as depression or anxiety, and may withdraw from social activities.

Middle-stage dementia is characterized by more severe cognitive decline and behavioral symptoms. The patient may have difficulty recognizing familiar people or places, and they may become disoriented or lost in familiar environments. They may also exhibit behavioral symptoms such as wandering, agitation, and aggression. In addition, the patient may have difficulty with personal care tasks, such as bathing, dressing, and grooming.

Late-stage dementia is characterized by severe cognitive decline and an increased dependence on caregivers. The patient may no longer be able to communicate verbally and may be confined to a wheelchair or bed. They may also experience difficulty swallowing and have an increased risk of infections and other complications.

In addition to memory loss and cognitive decline, there are other early warning signs of dementia that caregivers should be aware of. These can include changes in mood or personality, difficulty with language and communication, and problems with motor skills. The patient may also experience a loss of interest in activities that they previously enjoyed.

It is important to note that not all memory loss or cognitive decline is a sign of dementia. Many factors can contribute to memory loss and cognitive decline, including depression, medication side effects, and other medical conditions. However, if these symptoms persist and begin to interfere with daily activities, it is important to seek medical attention.

If you are concerned about yourself or a loved one, there are several steps you can take. The first step is to talk to your doctor. Your doctor can perform a variety of tests, including neurological and cognitive exams, blood tests, and brain imaging scans, to help determine if there is an underlying medical condition causing the symptoms.

In addition to medical intervention, there are also lifestyle changes that can help reduce the risk of developing dementia. Eating a healthy diet, exercising regularly, getting enough sleep, and staying socially active are all important for maintaining brain health. Additionally, avoiding smoking and excessive alcohol consumption can also help reduce the risk of developing dementia.

In conclusion, dementia is a progressive and degenerative condition that affects millions of people worldwide. Early diagnosis and management of the disease are crucial for ensuring the best possible outcomes for patients and their caregivers. The common symptoms and early warning signs of dementia include memory loss, cognitive decline, changes in mood or personality, difficulty with language and communication, and problems with motor skills. If you are concerned about yourself or a loved one, it is important to seek medical attention and make lifestyle changes that can help reduce the risk of developing dementia.

Some of the most common symptoms of dementia include:

- Memory loss, particularly short-term memory
- Difficulty with language and communication, including finding the right words
- Difficulty with problem-solving and decision-making
- Difficulty with spatial awareness and coordination
- Difficulty completing familiar tasks or following routines
- Changes in mood, personality, or behavior
- Confusion and disorientation, particularly with time and place
- Difficulty with judgment and reasoning
- Poor hygiene and self-care
- Loss of interest in hobbies and activities

- Social withdrawal and isolation
- Paranoia, delusions, or hallucinations (not always present)
- Changes in sleep patterns, such as sleeping during the day and being awake at night (not always present)
- Incontinence (not always present)

It is important to note that not all symptoms may be present in an individual with dementia, and that symptoms can vary widely from person to person. It is also essential to consult a healthcare professional for an accurate diagnosis and treatment plan.

Chapter Two

Causes and Risk Factors

Dementia is a complex condition that is caused by a variety of factors, including genetics, age, lifestyle, and environmental factors. It is a progressive and degenerative disease that affects memory, thinking, behavior, and emotions. Below we will we will explore the causes and risk factors of dementia.

One of the most significant risk factors for dementia is age. As people age, the risk of developing dementia increases. While dementia can affect people of all ages, it is most commonly associated with aging. It is estimated that the prevalence of dementia doubles every five years after the age of 65.

Genetics also plays a role in the development of dementia. While most cases of dementia are not directly caused by genetic factors, there are some genetic mutations that can increase the risk of developing the disease. For example, mutations in the genes that produce amyloid protein can increase the risk of developing Alzheimer's disease.

Lifestyle factors also play a significant role in the development of dementia. Poor diet, lack of exercise, smoking, and excessive alcohol consumption can all increase the risk of developing dementia. A healthy diet that is high in fruits, vegetables, whole grains, and lean protein can help reduce the risk of developing dementia. Exercise has also been shown to be beneficial for brain health and can help reduce the risk of developing dementia.

Environmental factors, such as exposure to toxins or pollutants, can also increase the risk of developing dementia. For example, exposure to pesticides has been linked to an increased risk of developing Parkinson's disease, which can also cause dementia. In addition, head injuries and trauma have been linked to an increased risk of developing dementia later in life.

There are several medical conditions that can increase the risk of developing dementia. Cardiovascular disease, diabetes, and high blood pressure can all contribute to the development of dementia. Additionally, untreated depression and anxiety can increase the risk of developing dementia.

There are also certain lifestyle factors that can increase the risk of developing specific types of dementia. For example, heavy alcohol consumption is a risk factor for Wernicke-Korsakoff syndrome, which is a type of dementia caused by a deficiency in thiamine. Smoking has also been linked to an increased risk of vascular dementia.

In conclusion, dementia is a complex condition that is caused by a variety of factors. Age, genetics, lifestyle factors, environmental factors, and medical conditions can all increase the risk of developing dementia. While there is no guaranteed way to prevent the development of dementia, making lifestyle changes that promote brain health can help reduce the risk of developing the disease. Eating a healthy diet, exercising regularly, avoiding smoking and excessive alcohol consumption, and staying socially active are all important for maintaining brain health and reducing the risk of developing dementia.

Neurodegenerative diseases and dementia

Dementia is a neurodegenerative disease that affects millions of people worldwide. Neurodegenerative diseases are a group of conditions that cause the progressive degeneration and death of neurons in the brain and nervous system. Below we will we will explore the relationship between neurodegenerative diseases and dementia.

There are several neurodegenerative diseases that can cause dementia, including Alzheimer's disease, Parkinson's disease, Huntington's disease, and Creutzfeldt-Jakob disease. Each of these diseases is characterized by the progressive degeneration and death of neurons in specific areas of the brain.

Alzheimer's disease is the most common cause of dementia, accounting for up to 70% of cases. It is a progressive and irreversible brain disease that affects memory, thinking, and behavior. Alzheimer's disease is characterized by the presence of amyloid plaques and neurofibrillary tangles in the brain, which are believed to contribute to the death of neurons.

Parkinson's disease is a progressive neurological disorder that can also cause dementia. It is caused by the degeneration of dopamine-producing neurons in the brain, which can lead to tremors, stiffness, and problems with movement. In addition to motor symptoms, Parkinson's disease can also cause cognitive impairment and dementia.

Huntington's disease is a genetic disorder that causes the progressive degeneration of neurons in the brain. It is characterized by the presence of abnormal protein deposits in the brain, which can lead to the death of neurons. Huntington's disease can cause a range of symptoms, including motor problems, cognitive decline, and behavioral changes.

Creutzfeldt-Jakob disease is a rare and fatal neurodegenerative disease that is caused by the accumulation of abnormal proteins in the brain. It can cause a range of symptoms, including dementia, muscle stiffness, and vision changes. Creutzfeldt-Jakob disease is often misdiagnosed as other neurological conditions, but it has its own unique set of symptoms and diagnostic criteria.

In addition to these specific neurodegenerative diseases, there are other conditions that can cause dementia, such as vascular dementia, which is caused by a reduction in blood flow to the brain, and Lewy body dementia, which is caused by abnormal protein deposits in the brain.

The exact cause of neurodegenerative diseases is not fully understood, but it is believed to be caused by a combination of genetic, environmental, and lifestyle factors. Age is also a significant risk factor for the development of neurodegenerative diseases, as the risk of developing these diseases increases with age.

There is currently no cure for neurodegenerative diseases, and treatment options are limited. However, there are several lifestyle changes that can help reduce the risk of developing these diseases, such as eating a healthy diet, exercising regularly, and avoiding smoking and excessive alcohol consumption.

Research into the causes and treatment of neurodegenerative diseases is ongoing, and new therapies and interventions are being developed. Early diagnosis and management of these diseases are crucial for ensuring the best possible outcomes for patients and their caregivers.

In conclusion, neurodegenerative diseases are a group of conditions that cause the progressive degeneration and death of neurons in the brain and nervous system. Dementia is a common symptom of many neurodegenerative diseases, including Alzheimer's disease, Parkinson's disease, Huntington's disease, and Creutzfeldt-Jakob disease. While the exact cause of these diseases is not fully understood, age, genetics, and lifestyle factors can all contribute to their development. Early diagnosis and management are crucial for ensuring the best possible outcomes for patients and their caregivers, and research into the causes and treatment of these diseases is ongoing.

Genetic and environmental factors

Dementia is a complex condition that is caused by a variety of factors, including genetics and environmental factors. It is a progressive and degenerative disease that affects memory, thinking, behavior, and emotions. Below we will we will explore the role of genetic and environmental factors in the development of dementia.

Genetics plays a significant role in the development of dementia. There are several genes that have been linked to an increased risk of developing the disease, including the APOE gene, which is associated with Alzheimer's disease. Individuals who carry certain genetic mutations have a higher risk of developing the disease than those who do not carry these mutations.

While genetics can play a role in the development of dementia, it is important to note that not all cases of dementia are directly caused by genetic factors. In fact, the majority of cases of dementia are caused by a combination of genetic, environmental, and lifestyle factors.

Environmental factors can also contribute to the development of dementia. Exposure to toxins or pollutants, such as lead or pesticides, can increase the risk of developing the disease. Additionally, head injuries and trauma have been linked to an increased risk of developing dementia later in life.

In addition to environmental factors, lifestyle factors can also play a significant role in the development of dementia. Poor diet, lack of exercise, smoking, and excessive alcohol consumption can all increase the risk of developing the disease. A healthy diet that is high in fruits, vegetables, whole grains, and lean protein can help reduce the risk of developing dementia. Exercise has also been shown to be beneficial for brain health and can help reduce the risk of developing dementia.

One of the most significant environmental factors that can contribute to the development of dementia is chronic stress. Chronic stress can cause changes in the brain that can lead to cognitive decline and an increased risk of developing dementia. Stress reduction techniques, such as meditation and mindfulness, can help reduce the risk of developing dementia.

It is important to note that not all environmental factors are modifiable. For example, air pollution and exposure to certain chemicals may be beyond an individual's control. However, making lifestyle changes that promote brain health can help reduce the risk of developing dementia.

While genetics and environmental factors can both contribute to the development of dementia, it is important to remember that the disease is complex and can be influenced by a variety of factors. Early diagnosis and management of the disease are crucial for ensuring the best possible outcomes for patients and their caregivers.

In conclusion, genetics and environmental factors both play a significant role in the development of dementia. While genetics can increase the risk of developing the disease, lifestyle factors such as poor diet, lack of exercise, smoking, and excessive alcohol consumption can also contribute to the development of the disease. Additionally, exposure to toxins or pollutants and chronic stress can also increase the risk of developing dementia. Making lifestyle changes that promote brain health can help reduce the risk of developing the disease, and early diagnosis and management are crucial for ensuring the best possible outcomes for patients and their caregivers.

Lifestyle choices and modifiable risks

Dementia is a complex condition that can be caused by a variety of factors, including genetics, age, and lifestyle choices. Lifestyle choices such as diet, exercise, smoking, and alcohol consumption can all contribute to the development of dementia. Below we will we will explore the role of lifestyle choices and modifiable risks in the development of dementia.

Diet is an important factor in maintaining brain health and reducing the risk of developing dementia. A healthy diet that is high in fruits, vegetables, whole grains, and lean protein can help reduce the risk of developing the disease. In addition, a diet that is low in saturated fats, processed foods, and sugar can also help reduce the risk of developing dementia. Studies have shown that the Mediterranean diet, which is high in fruits, vegetables, whole grains, and healthy fats, is particularly beneficial for brain health.

Exercise is another important lifestyle choice that can help reduce the risk of developing dementia. Regular exercise has been shown to improve cognitive function and reduce the risk of developing the disease. Exercise can also help reduce stress, which is a risk factor for dementia. A combination of aerobic exercise, such as running or cycling, and strength training, such as weightlifting or resistance training, is recommended for maintaining brain health.

Smoking is a modifiable risk factor for dementia. Smoking can cause damage to the blood vessels in the brain, which can lead to cognitive decline and an increased risk of developing the disease. Quitting smoking can help reduce the risk of developing dementia and improve overall health.

Excessive alcohol consumption is also a modifiable risk factor for dementia. Heavy drinking can cause damage to the brain and increase the risk of developing the disease. Limiting alcohol consumption to moderate levels, which is defined as one drink per day for women and two drinks per day for men, can help reduce the risk of developing dementia.

Chronic stress is a modifiable risk factor for dementia. Chronic stress can cause changes in the brain that can lead to cognitive decline and an increased risk of developing the disease. Stress reduction techniques, such as meditation and mindfulness, can help reduce the risk of developing dementia.

In addition to these lifestyle choices, managing medical conditions such as high blood pressure, diabetes, and depression can also help reduce the risk of developing dementia. These conditions can cause damage to the blood vessels in the brain, which can lead to cognitive decline and an increased risk of developing the disease. Managing these conditions through medication and lifestyle changes can help reduce the risk of developing dementia.

In conclusion, lifestyle choices such as diet, exercise, smoking, and alcohol consumption can all contribute to the development of dementia. Making healthy lifestyle choices, such as eating a healthy diet, exercising regularly, quitting smoking, limiting alcohol consumption, and reducing stress, can help reduce the risk of developing the disease. Managing medical conditions such as high blood pressure, diabetes, and depression can also help reduce the risk of developing dementia. Early diagnosis and management of the disease are crucial for ensuring the best possible outcomes for patients and their caregivers.

Chapter Three

Diagnosis and Assessment

Diagnosis and assessment of dementia is a complex process that requires a combination of medical and cognitive evaluations. Dementia is a progressive and degenerative disease that affects memory, thinking, behavior, and emotions. Below we will we will explore the process of diagnosis and assessment of dementia.

The first step in the diagnosis of dementia is a medical evaluation. A doctor will review the patient's medical history and perform a physical examination to rule out any underlying medical conditions that could be causing the symptoms. Blood tests may also be conducted to check for underlying medical conditions such as thyroid dysfunction or vitamin deficiencies.

Once medical conditions have been ruled out, a cognitive evaluation is performed to assess the patient's cognitive function. This typically involves a series of tests and assessments that evaluate memory, language, attention, and problem-solving abilities. The tests can include a Mini-Mental State Examination (MMSE), Montreal Cognitive Assessment (MoCA), and Clock Drawing Test.

Neuroimaging tests, such as magnetic resonance imaging (MRI) and positron emission tomography (PET) scans, may also be conducted to assess the structure and function of the brain. These tests can help rule out other conditions that can cause cognitive impairment, such as strokes or brain tumors.

The assessment process also involves evaluating the patient's functional abilities, including their ability to perform activities of daily living (ADLs) such as bathing, dressing, and grooming. This assessment can help determine the level of support and care that the patient may require.

It is important to note that the diagnosis and assessment of dementia can be challenging, as the symptoms can be subtle and may not be apparent in the early stages of the disease. Additionally, there can be a significant overlap in the symptoms of different types of dementia, making it difficult to distinguish between them.

There are several different types of dementia, each with its own unique set of symptoms and diagnostic criteria. Alzheimer's disease is the most common form of dementia, accounting for up to 70% of cases. Vascular dementia is another common form of dementia, which is caused by a reduction in blood flow to the brain.

Lewy body dementia is a type of dementia that is characterized by abnormal protein deposits in the brain. Frontotemporal dementia is a type of dementia that affects the frontal and temporal lobes of the brain, which are responsible for language and behavior. Parkinson's disease can also cause dementia, particularly in the later stages of the disease.

In conclusion, the diagnosis and assessment of dementia is a complex process that requires a combination of medical and cognitive evaluations. Medical evaluations are used to rule out underlying medical conditions, while cognitive evaluations are used to assess cognitive function. Neuroimaging tests can also be used to assess the structure and function of the brain. It is important to note that there are several different types of dementia, each with its own unique set of symptoms and diagnostic criteria. Early diagnosis and management of the disease are crucial for ensuring the best possible outcomes for patients and their caregivers.

The diagnostic process and tools

The diagnostic process for dementia involves a comprehensive evaluation of the patient's medical and cognitive history, as well as a range of assessments and tests to determine the cause and severity of the disease. Dementia is a complex and progressive disease that affects memory, thinking, behavior, and emotions. Below we will we will explore the diagnostic process and tools used in the diagnosis of dementia.

The diagnostic process for dementia typically begins with a medical evaluation, which involves a review of the patient's medical history, family history, and current medications. The doctor will also perform a physical examination to rule out any underlying medical conditions that could be causing the symptoms. Blood tests may also be conducted to check for underlying medical conditions such as thyroid dysfunction or vitamin deficiencies.

Once medical conditions have been ruled out, a cognitive evaluation is performed to assess the patient's cognitive function. This typically involves a series of tests and assessments that evaluate memory, language, attention, and problem-solving abilities. The tests can include a Mini-Mental State Examination (MMSE), Montreal Cognitive Assessment (MoCA), and Clock Drawing Test. The results of these tests are used to determine the severity and type of dementia.

Neuroimaging tests, such as magnetic resonance imaging (MRI) and positron emission tomography (PET) scans, may also be conducted to assess the structure and function of the brain. These tests can help rule out other conditions that can cause cognitive impairment, such as strokes or brain tumors.

There are several different types of dementia, each with its own unique set of symptoms and diagnostic criteria. Alzheimer's disease is the most common form of dementia, accounting for up to 70% of cases. Vascular dementia is another common form of dementia, which is caused by a reduction in blood flow to the brain.

Lewy body dementia is a type of dementia that is characterized by abnormal protein deposits in the brain. Frontotemporal dementia is a type of dementia that affects the frontal and temporal lobes of the brain, which are responsible for language and behavior. Parkinson's disease can also cause dementia, particularly in the later stages of the disease.

The diagnostic process for dementia can be challenging, as the symptoms can be subtle and may not be apparent in the early stages of the disease. Additionally, there can be a significant overlap in the symptoms of different types of dementia, making it difficult to distinguish between them.

In addition to the cognitive tests and neuroimaging tests, there are several other tools that can be used in the diagnosis of dementia. The Clinical Dementia Rating (CDR) is a tool that is used to assess the severity of dementia and determine the appropriate level of care. The Global Deterioration Scale (GDS) is a tool that is used to assess the stage of dementia and the level of impairment.

The Mini-Cog is a brief cognitive screening tool that can be used to assess memory and thinking skills. The Clock Drawing Test is another cognitive screening tool that is used to assess spatial and executive functioning.

In conclusion, the diagnostic process for dementia involves a comprehensive evaluation of the patient's medical and cognitive history, as well as a range of assessments and tests to determine the cause and severity of the disease. The process can be challenging, as there can be a significant overlap in the symptoms of different types of dementia. Neuroimaging tests, cognitive tests, and other diagnostic tools are used to aid in the diagnosis and assessment of dementia. Early diagnosis and management of the disease are crucial for ensuring the best possible outcomes for patients and their caregivers.

Differentiating between types of dementia

Dementia is a term that refers to a group of degenerative brain disorders that affect memory, thinking, behavior, and emotions. There are several different types of dementia, each with its own unique set of symptoms and diagnostic criteria. Below we will we will explore the differences between the different types of dementia.

Alzheimer's disease is the most common form of dementia, accounting for up to 70% of cases. It is a progressive disease that affects memory, thinking, and behavior. In the early stages of the disease, individuals may experience mild memory loss and difficulty with language and communication. As the disease progresses, individuals may have difficulty with activities of daily living and may experience changes in behavior and personality.

Vascular dementia is another common form of dementia, which is caused by a reduction in blood flow to the brain. It is the second most common type of dementia, accounting for up to 20% of cases. The symptoms of vascular dementia can vary depending on the location and severity of the damage to the brain. Individuals with vascular dementia may experience memory loss, difficulty with language and communication, and problems with motor coordination.

Lewy body dementia is a type of dementia that is characterized by abnormal protein deposits in the brain. It is the third most common form of dementia, accounting for up to 15% of cases. Individuals with Lewy body dementia may experience fluctuations in cognitive function, hallucinations, and difficulty with movement and balance.

Frontotemporal dementia is a type of dementia that affects the frontal and temporal lobes of the brain, which are responsible for language and behavior. It is a relatively rare form of dementia, accounting for up to 5% of cases. Individuals with frontotemporal dementia may experience changes in personality and behavior, as well as difficulty with language and communication.

Parkinson's disease can also cause dementia, particularly in the later stages of the disease. Individuals with Parkinson's disease dementia may experience difficulty with memory and thinking, as well as problems with movement and balance.

There are also several other less common forms of dementia, including Creutzfeldt-Jakob disease, Huntington's disease, and Wernicke-Korsakoff syndrome.

Differentiating between the different types of dementia can be challenging, as there can be a significant overlap in the symptoms of different types of dementia. It is important to note that some individuals may have more than one type of dementia, which can further complicate the diagnosis.

The diagnostic process for dementia typically involves a comprehensive evaluation of the patient's medical and cognitive history, as well as a range of assessments and tests to determine the cause and severity of the disease. Neuroimaging tests, such as magnetic resonance imaging (MRI) and positron emission tomography (PET) scans, may also be conducted to assess the structure and function of the brain.

In conclusion, there are several different types of dementia, each with its own unique set of symptoms and diagnostic criteria. Alzheimer's disease is the most common form of dementia, accounting for up to 70% of cases. Vascular dementia, Lewy body dementia, frontotemporal dementia, and Parkinson's disease dementia are other common types of dementia. Differentiating between the different types of dementia can be challenging, and a comprehensive evaluation of the patient's medical and cognitive history, as well as neuroimaging tests, are often used in the diagnosis and assessment of the disease. Early diagnosis and management of the disease are crucial for ensuring the best possible outcomes for patients and their caregivers.

The importance of early diagnosis

Dementia is a progressive and degenerative disease that affects memory, thinking, behavior, and emotions. It can have a significant impact on a person's quality of life, as well as the lives of their caregivers and loved ones. Early diagnosis of dementia is crucial for ensuring the best possible outcomes for patients and their caregivers. Below we will we will explore the importance of early diagnosis of dementia.

One of the primary reasons for the importance of early diagnosis is the fact that many of the symptoms of dementia can be caused by other medical conditions. Early diagnosis can help rule out underlying medical conditions that may be causing the symptoms, and ensure that the patient receives the appropriate treatment. For example, memory loss can be caused by conditions such as depression, vitamin deficiencies, and thyroid dysfunction.

Early diagnosis can also help ensure that the patient receives the appropriate treatment for their specific type of dementia. There are several different types of dementia, each with its own unique set of symptoms and diagnostic criteria. Alzheimer's disease is the most common form of dementia, accounting for up to 70% of cases. Vascular dementia, Lewy body dementia, frontotemporal dementia, and Parkinson's disease dementia are other common types of dementia. Different types of dementia may require different treatments and management strategies.

Early diagnosis can also help individuals with dementia and their caregivers plan for the future. It can help them understand what to expect and prepare for the changes that may occur as the disease progresses. This can include making important decisions about healthcare, finances, and living arrangements.

Another important reason for early diagnosis is that it allows individuals with dementia to participate in clinical trials and research studies. Clinical trials and research studies are crucial for advancing our understanding of the disease and developing new treatments and management strategies. Individuals with dementia who participate in these studies can play a vital role in helping to find a cure for the disease.

Early diagnosis also allows individuals with dementia to receive appropriate care and support. It can help ensure that they receive the appropriate level of care, and that their caregivers have access to the resources and support they need. This can include access to support groups, respite care, and other services that can help ease the burden of caregiving.

There are several different methods for diagnosing dementia, including medical evaluations, cognitive assessments, and neuroimaging tests. The diagnostic process can be challenging, as the symptoms of dementia can be subtle and may not be apparent in the early stages of the disease. However, early diagnosis is crucial for ensuring the best possible outcomes for patients and their caregivers.

In conclusion, early diagnosis of dementia is crucial for ensuring the best possible outcomes for patients and their caregivers. It allows for the appropriate treatment and management of the disease, helps individuals plan for the future, allows for participation in clinical trials and research studies, and ensures access to appropriate care and support. While the diagnostic process can be challenging, early diagnosis is essential for maximizing quality of life and improving outcomes for individuals with dementia and their caregivers.

Chapter Four

Treatment Options

Dementia is a progressive and degenerative disease that affects memory, thinking, behavior, and emotions. While there is currently no cure for dementia, there are several treatment options that can help manage the symptoms of the disease and improve quality of life for patients and their caregivers. Below we will we will explore the treatment options for dementia.

Pharmacological treatment is one of the primary treatment options for dementia. There are several medications that can help manage the symptoms of dementia, including cholinesterase inhibitors and memantine. Cholinesterase inhibitors, such as donepezil, rivastigmine, and galantamine, work by increasing the levels of acetylcholine in the brain, which can improve memory and thinking. Memantine is a medication that works by regulating glutamate, a neurotransmitter that is involved in learning and memory.

While these medications can help manage the symptoms of dementia, they are not a cure for the disease and do not slow down its progression. Additionally, these medications can have side effects, such as nausea, vomiting, and diarrhea.

Non-pharmacological treatments can also be effective in managing the symptoms of dementia. Cognitive stimulation therapy, music therapy, and art therapy are all examples of non-pharmacological treatments that can improve cognitive function and quality of life for patients with dementia.

Cognitive stimulation therapy involves engaging patients in a range of activities that stimulate cognitive function, such as puzzles, games, and group discussions. Music therapy involves using music to improve mood and reduce agitation, and has been shown to improve cognitive function in some patients with dementia. Art therapy involves using art as a form of expression and communication, and has been shown to improve mood and reduce anxiety in patients with dementia.

Environmental modifications can also be effective in managing the symptoms of dementia. This can include modifications to the patient's living environment, such as reducing clutter and increasing lighting, as well as modifications to the patient's daily routine, such as providing structured activities and routines.

Caregiver support is also an important aspect of treatment for dementia. Caregivers play a vital role in the management of dementia, and providing them with the appropriate support and resources can help ease the burden of caregiving and improve outcomes for patients. This can include access to respite care, support groups, and counseling services.

In addition to these treatment options, there are several lifestyle factors that can help manage the symptoms of dementia. Regular exercise, a healthy diet, and social engagement are all important for maintaining cognitive function and improving quality of life for patients with dementia.

In conclusion, while there is currently no cure for dementia, there are several treatment options that can help manage the symptoms of the disease and improve quality of life for patients and their caregivers. Pharmacological treatments, non-pharmacological treatments, environmental modifications, caregiver support, and lifestyle factors are all important aspects of treatment for dementia. While the effectiveness of these treatments can vary depending on the type and severity of the disease, early diagnosis and management of the disease are crucial for ensuring the best possible outcomes for patients and their caregivers.

Pharmacological treatments and medications

Dementia is a progressive and degenerative disease that affects memory, thinking, behavior, and emotions. While there is currently no cure for dementia, there are several pharmacological treatments and medications that can help manage the symptoms of the disease and improve quality of life for patients and their caregivers. Below we will we will explore the pharmacological treatments and medications for dementia.

1. Cholinesterase inhibitors are one of the primary medications used to treat dementia. These medications work by increasing the levels of acetylcholine in the brain, which is a neurotransmitter that is involved in memory and thinking. There are three main cholinesterase inhibitors used to treat dementia: donepezil, rivastigmine, and galantamine.

Donepezil is used to treat mild to moderate Alzheimer's disease. It is taken once a day and is available in tablet form. Rivastigmine is used to treat mild to moderate Alzheimer's disease and Parkinson's disease dementia. It is available in capsule and patch form. Galantamine is used to treat mild to moderate Alzheimer's disease. It is taken twice a day and is available in tablet and liquid form.

While these medications can help manage the symptoms of dementia, they are not a cure for the disease and do not slow down its progression. Additionally, these medications can have side effects, such as nausea, vomiting, and diarrhea.

Memantine is another medication used to treat dementia. It works by regulating glutamate, a neurotransmitter that is involved in learning and memory. Memantine is used to treat moderate to severe Alzheimer's disease, and is taken once a day in tablet form. Memantine can have side effects, such as headache, dizziness, and confusion.

Antidepressant medications are also sometimes used to treat depression and anxiety in patients with dementia. Selective serotonin reuptake inhibitors (SSRIs) and tricyclic antidepressants are the two main types of antidepressant medications used to treat depression and anxiety in patients with dementia.

SSRIs work by increasing the levels of serotonin in the brain, which is a neurotransmitter that is involved in mood regulation. Tricyclic antidepressants work by increasing the levels of norepinephrine and serotonin in the brain. These medications can have side effects, such as drowsiness, dry mouth, and constipation.

Antipsychotic medications are sometimes used to treat behavioral and psychological symptoms of dementia, such as aggression, agitation, and hallucinations. However, the use of antipsychotic medications in patients with dementia is controversial, as these medications can have serious side effects, such as an increased risk of stroke and mortality.

In conclusion, while there is currently no cure for dementia, there are several pharmacological treatments and medications that can help manage the symptoms of the disease and improve quality of life for patients and their caregivers. Cholinesterase inhibitors and memantine are the two main types of medications used to treat dementia. Antidepressant medications and antipsychotic medications may also be used to treat depression, anxiety, and behavioral symptoms in patients with dementia. While these medications can be effective in managing the symptoms of the disease, they are not a cure and can have side effects. It is important to work closely with a healthcare provider to determine the best treatment options for individuals with dementia.

Non-pharmacological approaches

Dementia is a progressive and degenerative disease that affects memory, thinking, behavior, and emotions. While there is currently no cure for dementia, there are several non-pharmacological approaches that can help manage the symptoms of the disease and improve quality of life for patients and their caregivers. Below we will we will explore the non-pharmacological approaches for dementia.

Cognitive stimulation therapy is a non-pharmacological approach that involves engaging patients in a range of activities that stimulate cognitive function. This can include puzzles, games, and group discussions. Cognitive stimulation therapy has been shown to improve cognitive function and quality of life for patients with dementia.

Music therapy is another non-pharmacological approach that can improve mood and reduce agitation in patients with dementia. Music therapy involves using music to stimulate the brain and promote relaxation. It has been shown to improve cognitive function in some patients with dementia.

Art therapy is another non-pharmacological approach that can improve mood and reduce anxiety in patients with dementia. Art therapy involves using art as a form of expression and communication. It can help patients with dementia express themselves and communicate their emotions, which can improve their quality of life.

Environmental modifications can also be effective in managing the symptoms of dementia. This can include modifications to the patient's living environment, such as reducing clutter and increasing lighting, as well as modifications to the patient's daily routine, such as providing structured activities and routines.

Caregiver support is also an important aspect of non-pharmacological treatment for dementia. Caregivers play a vital role in the management of dementia, and providing them with the appropriate support and resources can help ease the burden of caregiving and improve outcomes for patients. This can include access to respite care, support groups, and counseling services.

In addition to these non-pharmacological approaches, there are several lifestyle factors that can help manage the symptoms of dementia. Regular exercise, a healthy diet, and social engagement are all important for maintaining cognitive function and improving quality of life for patients with dementia.

In conclusion, while there is currently no cure for dementia, there are several non-pharmacological approaches that can help manage the symptoms of the disease and improve quality of life for patients and their caregivers. Cognitive stimulation therapy, music therapy, and art therapy are all effective non-pharmacological approaches for improving cognitive function and reducing symptoms of dementia. Environmental modifications, caregiver support, and lifestyle factors are also important aspects of non-pharmacological treatment for dementia. It is important to work closely with a healthcare provider to determine the best non-pharmacological approaches for individuals with dementia.

Emerging therapies and ongoing research

Dementia is a progressive and degenerative disease that affects memory, thinking, behavior, and emotions. While there is currently no cure for dementia, ongoing research is focused on developing new therapies that can improve outcomes for patients with the disease. Below we will we will explore some of the emerging therapies and ongoing research for dementia.

Immunotherapy is an emerging therapy that is being studied as a potential treatment for Alzheimer's disease, which is the most common form of dementia. Immunotherapy involves using antibodies to target and remove amyloid plaques from the brain, which are thought to contribute to the development of Alzheimer's disease. Several clinical trials are currently underway to evaluate the safety and efficacy of immunotherapy for Alzheimer's disease.

Gene therapy is another emerging therapy that is being studied for the treatment of dementia. Gene therapy involves modifying the genes responsible for producing amyloid and tau proteins, which are associated with the development of Alzheimer's disease. Several clinical trials are currently underway to evaluate the safety and efficacy of gene therapy for Alzheimer's disease.

Stem cell therapy is also being studied as a potential treatment for dementia. Stem cell therapy involves using stem cells to replace damaged or dead brain cells, which can improve cognitive function and slow down the progression of the disease. Several clinical trials are currently underway to evaluate the safety and efficacy of stem cell therapy for dementia.

In addition to these emerging therapies, ongoing research is focused on understanding the underlying mechanisms of dementia and identifying new targets for therapy. One area of research is focused on understanding the role of inflammation in the development of dementia. Chronic inflammation has been shown to contribute to the development of several chronic diseases, including Alzheimer's disease. Researchers are studying ways to target inflammation as a potential therapeutic approach for dementia.

Another area of research is focused on understanding the role of the gut microbiome in the development of dementia. The gut microbiome is the collection of bacteria, viruses, and fungi that live in the gastrointestinal tract. Emerging research suggests that changes in the gut microbiome can contribute to the development of several chronic diseases, including Alzheimer's disease. Researchers are studying ways to modify the gut microbiome as a potential therapeutic approach for dementia.

In conclusion, while there is currently no cure for dementia, ongoing research is focused on developing new therapies that can improve outcomes for patients with the disease. Immunotherapy, gene therapy, and stem cell therapy are all emerging therapies that are being studied for the treatment of dementia. Ongoing research is also focused on understanding the underlying mechanisms of dementia and identifying new targets for therapy, such as inflammation and the gut microbiome. While these therapies are still in the early stages of development, they hold promise for improving outcomes for patients with dementia in the future.

Chapter Five

Managing Symptoms

Dementia is a progressive and degenerative disease that affects memory, thinking, behavior, and emotions. While there is currently no cure for dementia, there are several ways to manage the symptoms of the disease and improve quality of life for patients and their caregivers. Below we will we will explore the various ways of managing the symptoms of dementia.

Managing cognitive symptoms is a key aspect of dementia care. Memory loss is a common symptom of dementia, and there are several ways to manage this symptom. One effective strategy is to use memory aids, such as calendars, to-do lists, and reminder notes. These aids can help patients remember important tasks and events. Cognitive stimulation therapy is another effective strategy for managing cognitive symptoms. This therapy involves engaging patients in a range of activities that stimulate cognitive function, such as puzzles, games, and group discussions.

Managing behavioral symptoms is another important aspect of dementia care. Agitation, aggression, and wandering are common behavioral symptoms of dementia. There are several strategies for managing these symptoms, including environmental modifications, such as reducing noise and clutter, and providing structured activities and routines. Additionally, some medications, such as antipsychotics, can be used to manage behavioral symptoms. However, the use of antipsychotics in patients with dementia is controversial, as these medications can have serious side effects.

Managing emotional symptoms is also important in dementia care. Depression and anxiety are common emotional symptoms of dementia. Non-pharmacological approaches, such as music therapy and art therapy, can be effective in improving mood and reducing anxiety in patients with dementia. Antidepressant medications may also be used to treat depression and anxiety in patients with dementia.

Managing physical symptoms is another aspect of dementia care. Patients with dementia are at an increased risk of falls and injuries. Regular exercise, such as walking or swimming, can help improve strength and balance, and reduce the risk of falls. Additionally, it is important to ensure that patients with dementia receive adequate nutrition and hydration, as they may forget to eat or drink.

Managing sleep disturbances is another important aspect of dementia care. Patients with dementia often experience disrupted sleep patterns, which can lead to fatigue and daytime drowsiness. There are several strategies for managing sleep disturbances, such as creating a calm and relaxing sleeping environment, establishing a regular sleep routine, and reducing daytime napping.

In conclusion, while there is currently no cure for dementia, there are several ways to manage the symptoms of the disease and improve quality of life for patients and their caregivers. Managing cognitive symptoms, behavioral symptoms, emotional symptoms, physical symptoms, and sleep disturbances are all important aspects of dementia care. It is important to work closely with a healthcare provider to determine the best strategies for managing the symptoms of dementia. Additionally, providing adequate support and resources for caregivers is important in ensuring the best outcomes for patients with dementia.

Quick tips:

- Establish a daily routine and stick to it.
- Simplify the living environment to reduce confusion.
- Use labels and signs to help with orientation.
- Encourage physical exercise and activity to improve overall health.
- Provide a healthy and balanced diet.
- Ensure that medication is taken as prescribed.
- Use memory aids, such as calendars, clocks, and pill dispensers.
- Encourage socialization and interaction with others.
- Practice good communication techniques, such as speaking slowly and clearly.
- Monitor and manage challenging behaviors, such as aggression or wandering.
- Use music or other forms of sensory stimulation to soothe and calm.
- Provide opportunities for engagement and meaningful activities.
- Create a supportive and positive environment.
- Provide regular opportunities for rest and relaxation.
- Use assistive devices as needed, such as walkers or hearing aids.
- Consider alternative therapies, such as aromatherapy or massage.
- Monitor and manage any comorbid conditions, such as depres-

sion or anxiety.

- Encourage participation in support groups for individuals with dementia and their caregivers.
- Use technology to assist with memory and other cognitive functions.
- Monitor and minimize triggers for challenging behaviors.
- Provide regular opportunities for outdoor activities and exposure to natural light.
- Use humor and positive reinforcement to reduce stress and anxiety.
- Involve the individual with dementia in decision-making as much as possible.
- Monitor and manage sleep disturbances, such as insomnia or excessive sleepiness.
- Provide regular opportunities for intellectual stimulation and brain exercises.
- Consider the use of medication to manage symptoms, such as anxiety or depression.
- Use relaxation techniques, such as deep breathing or visualization exercises.
- Provide regular opportunities for creative expression, such as art or music therapy.
- Use reminiscence therapy to help with memory and mood.

- Ensure that the individual with dementia receives regular medical check-ups and evaluations.

Behavioral and psychological symptoms

Dementia is a progressive and degenerative disease that affects memory, thinking, behavior, and emotions. As the disease progresses, patients may experience a range of behavioral and psychological symptoms that can be challenging for both patients and caregivers. Below we will we will explore the behavioral and psychological symptoms of dementia and their management.

Agitation and aggression are common behavioral symptoms of dementia. Patients may become agitated or aggressive due to confusion, fear, or frustration. Environmental modifications, such as reducing noise and clutter, can be effective in reducing agitation and aggression. Additionally, providing structured activities and routines can help reduce boredom and frustration, which can contribute to agitation and aggression. Medications, such as antipsychotics, may also be used to manage agitation and aggression in some cases.

Wandering is another common behavioral symptom of dementia. Patients may wander due to confusion or a desire to explore. Environmental modifications, such as installing door locks or alarms, can be effective in reducing wandering. Additionally, providing structured activities and routines can help reduce boredom and restlessness, which can contribute to wandering.

Depression and anxiety are common psychological symptoms of dementia. Patients may experience depression and anxiety due to a sense of loss and confusion. Non-pharmacological approaches, such as music therapy and art therapy, can be effective in improving mood and reducing anxiety in patients with dementia. Antidepressant medications may also be used to treat depression and anxiety in patients with dementia.

Sleep disturbances are another common psychological symptom of dementia. Patients may experience disrupted sleep patterns, such as frequent waking or daytime drowsiness. Creating a calm and relaxing sleeping environment, establishing a regular sleep routine, and reducing daytime napping can be effective in managing sleep disturbances in patients with dementia.

Hallucinations and delusions are also common psychological symptoms of dementia. Patients may experience hallucinations and delusions due to changes in the brain. Medications, such as antipsychotics, may be used to manage hallucinations and delusions in some cases. However, the use of antipsychotics in patients with dementia is controversial, as these medications can have serious side effects.

Incontinence is a common behavioral symptom of dementia. Patients may experience urinary or fecal incontinence due to a loss of bladder or bowel control. Providing regular toilet breaks, using incontinence products, and maintaining good hygiene can be effective in managing incontinence in patients with dementia.

In conclusion, the behavioral and psychological symptoms of dementia can be challenging for both patients and caregivers. Agitation, aggression, wandering, depression, anxiety, sleep disturbances, hallucinations, delusions, and incontinence are all common symptoms of dementia. Environmental modifications, structured activities and routines, non-pharmacological approaches, and medications are all strategies that can be used to manage these symptoms. It is important to work closely with a healthcare provider to determine the best strategies for managing the behavioral and psychological symptoms of dementia. Additionally, providing adequate support and resources for caregivers is important in ensuring the best outcomes for patients with dementia.

Communication strategies

Communication is an important aspect of dementia care, as patients may experience changes in language and communication skills as the disease progresses. Patients with dementia may experience difficulty finding the right words, following conversations, and understanding complex sentences. Below we will we will explore communication strategies for patients with dementia.

One effective communication strategy for patients with dementia is to use simple and clear language. Using short and simple sentences can help patients better understand what is being said. Additionally, it is important to speak slowly and clearly, and to give patients time to process what has been said.

Another effective communication strategy is to use visual aids. Using pictures, diagrams, and gestures can help patients better understand what is being said. Additionally, it is important to maintain eye contact and use a friendly and reassuring tone of voice when communicating with patients with dementia.

Repeating key points and using a consistent message can also be effective in communicating with patients with dementia. Patients may experience difficulty retaining information, so repeating key points can help reinforce important information. Additionally, using a consistent message can help reduce confusion and improve understanding.

Active listening is another important aspect of communication with patients with dementia. Listening carefully to patients and providing feedback can help improve communication and build trust. Additionally, it is important to be patient and understanding when communicating with patients with dementia, and to avoid correcting or criticizing their speech.

It is also important to pay attention to nonverbal cues when communicating with patients with dementia. Patients may communicate their needs and emotions through nonverbal cues, such as facial expressions, body language, and tone of voice. Paying attention to these cues can help improve communication and better understand the patient's needs.

Finally, it is important to consider the environment when communicating with patients with dementia. Patients may experience difficulty focusing and understanding in noisy or cluttered environments. Creating a quiet and calm environment can help improve communication and reduce frustration and confusion.

In conclusion, communication is an important aspect of dementia care. Patients with dementia may experience difficulty finding the right words, following conversations, and understanding complex sentences. Using simple and clear language, visual aids, repeating key points, active listening, paying attention to nonverbal cues, and considering the environment are all effective communication strategies for patients with dementia. It is important to work closely with a healthcare provider to determine the best strategies for communicating with patients with dementia. Additionally, providing adequate support and resources for caregivers is important in ensuring the best outcomes for patients with dementia.

Coping with memory loss

Memory loss is a common symptom of dementia, and can be challenging for both patients and caregivers. Coping with memory loss is an important aspect of dementia care, and there are several strategies that can help patients and caregivers better manage this symptom. Below we will we will explore strategies for coping with memory loss in patients with dementia.

One effective strategy for coping with memory loss is to use memory aids. Memory aids, such as calendars, to-do lists, and reminder notes, can help patients remember important tasks and events. Additionally, it is important to keep a consistent routine and schedule, as this can help reduce confusion and improve memory.

Creating a memory-friendly environment is another effective strategy for coping with memory loss. This involves reducing clutter and distractions in the environment, and using visual cues, such as labels and color-coded items, to help patients better remember where things are located. Additionally, it is important to use a consistent and organized layout in the environment, as this can help reduce confusion and improve memory.

Encouraging regular exercise and physical activity is also important in coping with memory loss. Regular exercise can help improve blood flow to the brain, which can improve memory and cognitive function. Additionally, engaging in mentally stimulating activities, such as puzzles, games, and social activities, can help improve memory and cognitive function.

Maintaining good nutrition and hydration is also important in coping with memory loss. Patients with dementia may forget to eat or drink, so it is important to provide regular meals and snacks, and to encourage patients to drink water and other fluids throughout the day.

It is also important to provide emotional support for patients with dementia. Memory loss can be frustrating and challenging for patients, and may lead to feelings of anxiety and depression. Providing emotional support, such as reassurance and encouragement, can help patients cope with memory loss and maintain a positive outlook.

Finally, it is important to involve caregivers in coping with memory loss. Caregivers play a crucial role in supporting patients with dementia, and may need to provide assistance with memory aids, creating a memory-friendly environment, and encouraging exercise and physical activity. It is important to provide caregivers with adequate support and resources, such as respite care and counseling services, to help them better manage the challenges of caring for a patient with dementia.

In conclusion, coping with memory loss is an important aspect of dementia care. Memory aids, creating a memory-friendly environment, regular exercise and physical activity, good nutrition and hydration, emotional support, and involving caregivers are all effective strategies for coping with memory loss in patients with dementia. It is important to work closely with a healthcare provider and provide adequate support and resources for caregivers in order to ensure the best outcomes for patients with dementia.

Chapter Six

Daily Living and Care

Daily living and care for patients with dementia can be challenging, as the disease can impact the patient's ability to perform basic activities of daily living, such as eating, bathing, dressing, and toileting. Additionally, patients with dementia may experience behavioral and psychological symptoms that can make daily living and care more difficult. Below we will we will explore strategies for daily living and care for patients with dementia.

One effective strategy for daily living and care is to create a structured routine. Patients with dementia may benefit from a consistent and structured daily routine that includes regular mealtimes, bathing and grooming, and social activities. Additionally, providing patients with visual cues, such as a written schedule or picture prompts, can help them better understand and follow the routine.

Creating a safe and secure environment is also important in daily living and care for patients with dementia. Patients with dementia may experience confusion and disorientation, which can increase the risk of falls and accidents. Ensuring that the environment is well-lit, free from clutter, and has adequate safety features, such as grab bars and non-slip mats, can help reduce the risk of accidents.

Encouraging independence and self-care is also important in daily living and care for patients with dementia. Patients with dementia may experience a loss of independence and a sense of helplessness, which can contribute to depression and anxiety. Encouraging patients to participate in self-care activities, such as dressing and grooming, and providing assistance when needed, can help maintain their sense of independence and dignity.

Managing nutrition and hydration is also important in daily living and care for patients with dementia. Patients with dementia may experience difficulty with eating and drinking, which can lead to dehydration and malnutrition. Providing regular meals and snacks, and ensuring that patients have access to water and other fluids throughout the day, can help prevent dehydration and malnutrition.

Managing incontinence is another important aspect of daily living and care for patients with dementia. Patients with dementia may experience urinary or fecal incontinence due to a loss of bladder or bowel control. Providing regular toilet breaks, using incontinence products, and maintaining good hygiene can be effective in managing incontinence in patients with dementia.

Finally, it is important to provide emotional support for patients with dementia and their caregivers. Daily living and care can be challenging for both patients and caregivers, and may lead to feelings of stress, frustration, and isolation. Providing emotional support, such as reassurance and encouragement, can help patients and caregivers cope with the challenges of daily living and care.

In conclusion, daily living and care for patients with dementia can be challenging, but there are effective strategies that can be used to improve outcomes. Creating a structured routine, creating a safe and secure environment, encouraging independence and self-care, managing nutrition and hydration, managing incontinence, and providing emotional support are all important aspects of daily living and care for patients with dementia. It is important to work closely with a healthcare provider and provide adequate support and resources for caregivers in order to ensure the best outcomes for patients with dementia.

Maintaining a safe and supportive environment

Maintaining a safe and supportive environment is an important aspect of dementia care, as patients with dementia may experience confusion, disorientation, and difficulty with memory and perception. A safe and supportive environment can help reduce the risk of accidents and falls, improve quality of life, and promote independence and autonomy. Below we will we will explore strategies for maintaining a safe and supportive environment for patients with dementia.

Creating a familiar and structured environment is an effective strategy for maintaining a safe and supportive environment. Patients with dementia may experience confusion and disorientation in unfamiliar environments, so it is important to create an environment that is familiar and consistent. Using familiar objects and furniture, such as family photos or favorite chairs, can help patients feel more comfortable and secure. Additionally, creating a structured routine and providing visual cues, such as written schedules or picture prompts, can help patients better understand and navigate their environment.

Ensuring that the environment is free from hazards and potential dangers is another important aspect of maintaining a safe and supportive environment. Patients with dementia may experience difficulty with perception and may be more prone to accidents and falls. Ensuring that the environment is well-lit, free from clutter, and has adequate safety features, such as grab bars and non-slip mats, can help reduce the risk of accidents and falls.

Providing regular exercise and physical activity is also important in maintaining a safe and supportive environment. Regular exercise can help improve strength, balance, and mobility, which can reduce the risk of accidents and falls. Additionally, engaging in mentally stimulating activities, such as puzzles and games, can help improve cognitive function and promote independence and autonomy.

Creating a supportive social environment is also important in maintaining a safe and supportive environment. Patients with dementia may experience feelings of loneliness and isolation, which can contribute to depression and anxiety. Creating opportunities for socialization, such as through group activities or visits from family and friends, can help improve quality of life and promote emotional well-being.

Managing medication and other medical needs is also important in maintaining a safe and supportive environment. Patients with dementia may experience difficulty with managing their medication and other medical needs, which can lead to complications and adverse events. Ensuring that medication is stored and administered correctly, and that patients receive regular medical care and attention, can help prevent medical complications and promote well-being.

Finally, it is important to provide emotional support for patients with dementia and their caregivers. Maintaining a safe and supportive environment can be challenging for both patients and caregivers, and may lead to feelings of stress, frustration, and isolation. Providing emotional support, such as reassurance and encouragement, can help patients and caregivers cope with the challenges of maintaining a safe and supportive environment.

In conclusion, maintaining a safe and supportive environment is an important aspect of dementia care. Creating a familiar and structured environment, ensuring that the environment is free from hazards and potential dangers, providing regular exercise and physical activity, creating a supportive social environment, managing medication and other medical needs, and providing emotional support are all important strategies for maintaining a safe and supportive environment for patients with dementia. It is important to work closely with a healthcare provider and provide adequate support and resources for caregivers in order to ensure the best outcomes for patients with dementia.

Assistive devices and technology

Assistive devices and technology can play an important role in improving the quality of life and independence for patients with dementia. These devices and technologies can help patients with dementia to perform daily activities, manage medical needs, and maintain social connections. Below we will we will explore some of the assistive devices and technologies available for patients with dementia.

One type of assistive device that can be helpful for patients with dementia is a mobility aid. Patients with dementia may experience difficulty with mobility and balance, which can increase the risk of accidents and falls. Mobility aids, such as walkers or canes, can help patients maintain their balance and independence. Additionally, devices such as lift chairs or stair lifts can help patients navigate their environment more easily and safely.

Assistive technologies can also be helpful for patients with dementia. For example, GPS devices can help patients with dementia who are at risk of wandering to be located quickly if they become lost. Medication reminders, such as electronic pill dispensers or reminder apps, can help patients manage their medication more effectively. Additionally, telehealth technologies, such as video conferencing with healthcare providers, can help patients access medical care and support more easily.

Environmental modifications can also be used as assistive devices for patients with dementia. Simple modifications, such as installing grab bars in the bathroom or using non-slip mats, can help reduce the risk of falls and accidents. Smart home technologies, such as sensors that detect motion or door sensors that alert caregivers when a patient has left the house, can help patients remain safe and independent while living at home.

Assistive devices and technology can also be used to support cognitive function and communication in patients with dementia. Devices such as memory aids, such as digital photo frames or memory books, can help patients remember important information, such as names or appointments. Assistive communication technologies, such as speech-to-text software or communication boards, can help patients with dementia communicate more effectively with their caregivers and healthcare providers.

Finally, assistive devices and technology can be used to promote social connections and engagement for patients with dementia. Devices such as social robots or virtual reality systems can provide patients with opportunities for social interaction and engagement, even if they are unable to leave their homes or communities. Additionally, video chat technologies, such as Skype or FaceTime, can help patients stay connected with their family and friends.

In conclusion, assistive devices and technology can play an important role in improving the quality of life and independence for patients with dementia. Mobility aids, assistive technologies, environmental modifications, cognitive and communication devices, and social engagement technologies are all available options for patients with dementia. It is important to work closely with a healthcare provider to identify which assistive devices and technologies are most appropriate for each patient's individual needs. Additionally, providing training and support for patients and caregivers on how to use these devices and technologies can help ensure their effectiveness and success.

Nutrition and hydration considerations

Nutrition and hydration are important considerations for patients with dementia. Patients with dementia may experience difficulty with eating and drinking, and may be at increased risk for malnutrition and dehydration. Below we will we will explore some of the nutrition and hydration considerations for patients with dementia.

One important consideration for patients with dementia is ensuring that they receive adequate hydration. Patients with dementia may experience difficulty with drinking, may forget to drink, or may not recognize when they are thirsty. Additionally, some medications used to treat dementia may increase the risk of dehydration. Ensuring that patients have access to fluids throughout the day, such as by providing water or juice in a favorite cup or mug, can help promote hydration.

Another important consideration is ensuring that patients with dementia receive a balanced and nutritious diet. Patients with dementia may experience difficulty with eating, may forget to eat, or may become disinterested in food. Ensuring that meals are presented in an appetizing and appealing manner, providing finger foods or foods that are easy to eat, and using familiar and favorite foods can help promote appetite and improve nutritional intake.

It is also important to consider any special dietary needs or restrictions for patients with dementia. Some patients with dementia may have difficulty chewing or swallowing, which can make it difficult to eat certain foods. Additionally, patients with dementia may have medical conditions, such as diabetes or high blood pressure, that require special dietary considerations.

Working closely with a healthcare provider and a registered dietitian can help ensure that patients with dementia receive a nutritionally balanced and appropriate diet.

Providing a supportive and calm dining environment is also important for patients with dementia. Patients with dementia may become agitated or anxious during meal times, which can make it difficult for them to eat. Providing a calm and quiet environment, minimizing distractions, and using familiar and comforting cues, such as playing soft music or using a favorite tablecloth, can help promote a relaxed and enjoyable dining experience.

Finally, it is important to consider any cultural or personal preferences when providing nutrition and hydration for patients with dementia. Patients with dementia may have specific cultural or personal preferences regarding food and drink, which should be taken into consideration. Additionally, involving patients in the meal planning and preparation process, such as by allowing them to choose their own meals or assist with cooking, can help promote a sense of autonomy and independence.

In conclusion, nutrition and hydration are important considerations for patients with dementia. Ensuring that patients receive adequate hydration, a balanced and nutritious diet, and a supportive dining environment can help promote overall health and well-being. Working closely with a healthcare provider and a registered dietitian can help ensure that patients with dementia receive appropriate and individualized nutrition and hydration care.

Chapter Seven

Physical Health and Dementia

Dementia is a neurodegenerative disease that affects cognitive function, memory, and behavior. However, dementia can also have significant effects on physical health. Patients with dementia may experience difficulty with mobility, balance, and self-care, which can increase the risk of falls and other physical health complications. Below we will we will explore the relationship between physical health and dementia.

One important aspect of physical health for patients with dementia is maintaining mobility and independence. Patients with dementia may experience difficulty with balance, coordination, and movement, which can increase the risk of falls and other injuries. Physical therapy and exercise programs can help patients maintain mobility and strength, reduce the risk of falls, and improve overall physical health. Additionally, mobility aids, such as walkers or canes, can help patients maintain their balance and independence.

Another important aspect of physical health for patients with dementia is maintaining good oral health. Patients with dementia may experience difficulty with brushing their teeth or may forget to do so, which can increase the risk of dental problems such as gum disease or tooth decay. Additionally, poor oral health can lead to other physical health complications such as pneumonia. Providing support and reminders for patients to brush their teeth and maintaining regular dental check-ups can help promote good oral health.

It is also important to consider nutrition and hydration for patients with dementia as part of their physical health care. Patients with dementia may experience difficulty with eating or may forget to eat, which can lead to malnutrition and other physical health complications. Ensuring that patients receive a balanced and nutritious diet, and that they are adequately hydrated, can help promote overall physical health.

Finally, it is important to consider the management of other medical conditions in patients with dementia. Patients with dementia may have other medical conditions, such as diabetes, high blood pressure, or heart disease, which require ongoing management. It is important to work closely with healthcare providers to ensure that patients with dementia receive appropriate and individualized care for these medical conditions.

In conclusion, physical health is an important consideration for patients with dementia. Maintaining mobility and independence, good oral health, proper nutrition and hydration, and the management of other medical conditions are all important aspects of physical health care for patients with dementia. Working closely with healthcare providers, including physical therapists, dentists, and registered dietitians, can help ensure that patients receive appropriate and individualized physical health care.

Exercise and mobility

Exercise and mobility are important considerations for patients with dementia. Dementia can affect a patient's physical abilities, leading to a decline in mobility, balance, and strength. However, regular exercise and physical activity can help maintain and improve physical function in patients with dementia. Below we will we will explore the importance of exercise and mobility for patients with dementia.

One important aspect of exercise and mobility for patients with dementia is maintaining independence. Patients with dementia may experience difficulty with movement, which can increase the risk of falls and other injuries. Physical therapy and exercise programs can help patients maintain mobility and strength, reduce the risk of falls, and improve overall physical health. Additionally, mobility aids, such as walkers or canes, can help patients maintain their balance and independence.

Exercise has also been shown to have cognitive benefits for patients with dementia. Regular exercise has been associated with improved cognitive function, including memory and attention, in patients with dementia. Exercise can also help improve mood and reduce the risk of depression, which is common in patients with dementia.

It is important to note that exercise and physical activity do not have to be strenuous or time-consuming. Simple activities, such as walking, gardening, or chair exercises, can have significant benefits for patients with dementia. Additionally, incorporating exercise into daily routines, such as taking a walk after meals or participating in group exercise classes, can help patients with dementia stay motivated and engaged.

Another important consideration is maintaining safe and appropriate exercise routines for patients with dementia. Patients with dementia may not be able to follow complex instructions or may forget how to perform certain exercises. Additionally, patients may have medical conditions that require specific modifications to exercise routines. It is important to work closely with healthcare providers and physical therapists to develop safe and appropriate exercise programs for patients with dementia.

Finally, it is important to consider the social benefits of exercise and mobility for patients with dementia. Exercise and physical activity can provide opportunities for social interaction and engagement, which can help reduce feelings of isolation and loneliness in patients with dementia. Group exercise classes or other social activities can help promote a sense of community and connectedness for patients with dementia.

In conclusion, exercise and mobility are important considerations for patients with dementia. Regular exercise can help maintain and improve physical function, cognitive function, and mood in patients with dementia. It is important to develop safe and appropriate exercise routines, incorporating simple activities and modifications as needed. Additionally, exercise and physical activity can provide important social benefits for patients with dementia, promoting a sense of community and connectedness.

Sleep and dementia

Sleep is an important aspect of overall health and well-being. However, for patients with dementia, sleep disturbances are common and can have significant negative effects on cognitive function, behavior, and quality of life. Below we will we will explore the relationship between sleep and dementia, including the causes and effects of sleep disturbances in patients with dementia.

One common sleep disturbance in patients with dementia is insomnia. Insomnia can manifest as difficulty falling asleep, staying asleep, or waking up too early. Insomnia can be caused by a variety of factors, including pain, anxiety, depression, and medication side effects. Additionally, changes in the sleep-wake cycle, or circadian rhythm, can contribute to insomnia in patients with dementia.

Another common sleep disturbance in patients with dementia is excessive daytime sleepiness. Patients with dementia may experience daytime sleepiness as a result of disrupted nighttime sleep or as a symptom of the underlying disease. Excessive daytime sleepiness can lead to decreased cognitive function, mood disturbances, and increased risk of falls and other injuries.

Sleep disturbances in patients with dementia can have significant negative effects on cognitive function. Sleep plays an important role in memory consolidation and cognitive function, and disruptions to sleep can lead to impaired cognitive function and memory problems. Additionally, sleep disturbances can exacerbate other behavioral symptoms of dementia, such as agitation and aggression.

There are a variety of interventions that can be used to address sleep disturbances in patients with dementia. Non-pharmacological interventions, such as behavioral therapies and sleep hygiene education, can be effective in promoting healthy sleep habits and improving sleep quality. Additionally, pharmacological interventions, such as sleep aids or medication adjustments, may be necessary for some patients with severe sleep disturbances.

It is important to note that treating sleep disturbances in patients with dementia can have important benefits beyond improved sleep quality. Addressing sleep disturbances can lead to improvements in cognitive function, mood, and behavior, as well as decreased risk of falls and other injuries.

In conclusion, sleep disturbances are common in patients with dementia and can have significant negative effects on cognitive function, behavior, and quality of life. Addressing sleep disturbances through a combination of non-pharmacological and pharmacological interventions can lead to significant improvements in sleep quality and overall well-being for patients with dementia. It is important for healthcare providers and caregivers to recognize the importance of sleep in patients with dementia and to work together to address sleep disturbances and promote healthy sleep habits.

Managing comorbid conditions

Dementia is a complex and multifaceted disease that often coexists with other medical conditions, known as comorbidities. Comorbid conditions can complicate the management of dementia, leading to increased healthcare needs, decreased quality of life, and increased healthcare costs. Below we will we will explore the management of comorbid conditions in patients with dementia, including the challenges and considerations for healthcare providers.

One common comorbid condition in patients with dementia is depression. Depression is common in patients with dementia and can exacerbate cognitive and behavioral symptoms. Depression can also complicate the management of dementia by decreasing adherence to medication regimens and increasing the risk of adverse health outcomes. Management of depression in patients with dementia may include medication, psychotherapy, or behavioral interventions.

Another common comorbid condition in patients with dementia is cardiovascular disease. Cardiovascular disease is a significant risk factor for cognitive decline and dementia, and patients with dementia are at increased risk for cardiovascular disease. Management of cardiovascular disease in patients with dementia may include medication, lifestyle modifications, and regular monitoring of blood pressure and cholesterol levels.

Diabetes is another common comorbid condition in patients with dementia. Diabetes can complicate the management of dementia by increasing the risk of cognitive decline and other health complications. Management of diabetes in patients with dementia may include medication, lifestyle modifications, and regular monitoring of blood glucose levels.

It is important to note that management of comorbid conditions in patients with dementia can be challenging due to the complex interplay between multiple medical conditions. Additionally, medications used to treat comorbid conditions may interact with medications used to treat dementia, leading to increased risk of adverse health outcomes. Healthcare providers must work closely together to develop comprehensive treatment plans that consider the potential interactions between medications and comorbid conditions.

Finally, it is important to consider the impact of comorbid conditions on the caregiver burden in patients with dementia. Caregivers of patients with dementia may experience increased stress and burden when managing comorbid conditions, leading to decreased quality of life and increased risk of burnout. It is important to provide caregivers with support and resources to manage the complex needs of patients with dementia and comorbid conditions.

In conclusion, managing comorbid conditions in patients with dementia is a complex and multifaceted task. Comorbid conditions, such as depression, cardiovascular disease, and diabetes, can complicate the management of dementia and lead to increased healthcare needs and decreased quality of life. Healthcare providers must work closely together to develop comprehensive treatment plans that consider the potential interactions between medications and comorbid conditions. Additionally, providing support and resources to caregivers is essential for managing the complex needs of patients with dementia and comorbid conditions.

Chapter Eight

Emotional Well-being and Mental Health

Emotional well-being and mental health are essential aspects of overall health and quality of life. In patients with dementia, emotional well-being and mental health can be significantly impacted by the disease and its associated symptoms. Below we will we will explore the relationship between dementia and emotional well-being and mental health, including the challenges and considerations for healthcare providers.

One common emotional symptom of dementia is depression. Depression is common in patients with dementia and can exacerbate cognitive and behavioral symptoms. Depression can also complicate the management of dementia by decreasing adherence to medication regimens and increasing the risk of adverse health outcomes. Management of depression in patients with dementia may include medication, psychotherapy, or behavioral interventions.

Another common emotional symptom of dementia is anxiety. Anxiety can manifest as restlessness, agitation, or fear, and can significantly impact quality of life for patients with dementia. Anxiety can be caused by a variety of factors, including medication side effects, changes in the environment, or fear of the disease and its progression. Management of anxiety in patients with dementia may include medication, behavioral interventions, or modifications to the environment to promote feelings of safety and security.

Additionally, behavioral symptoms such as aggression and agitation can significantly impact emotional well-being and mental health in patients with dementia. These symptoms can lead to increased caregiver burden and decreased quality of life for both patients and caregivers. Management of behavioral symptoms in patients with dementia may include medication, behavioral interventions, or modifications to the environment to promote feelings of safety and security.

It is important to note that emotional well-being and mental health can also impact the progression of dementia. Patients with poor emotional well-being and mental health may experience more rapid cognitive decline and increased risk of adverse health outcomes. Healthcare providers must consider the impact of emotional well-being and mental health on the progression of dementia and work to manage emotional symptoms and promote positive mental health.

Finally, it is important to consider the impact of dementia on caregiver emotional well-being and mental health. Caregivers of patients with dementia may experience increased stress and burden when managing emotional symptoms and behavioral disturbances, leading to decreased quality of life and increased risk of burnout. It is important to provide caregivers with support and resources to manage the emotional needs of patients with dementia and to promote their own emotional well-being and mental health.

In conclusion, emotional well-being and mental health are essential aspects of overall health and quality of life for patients with dementia. Emotional symptoms, such as depression and anxiety, as well as behavioral symptoms, such as aggression and agitation, can significantly impact quality of life for patients and caregivers. Healthcare providers must work to manage emotional symptoms and promote positive mental health in patients with dementia, while also considering the impact of emotional well-being and mental health on the progression of the disease. Additionally, providing support and resources to caregivers is essential for managing the emotional needs of patients with dementia and promoting caregiver well-being.

Depression and anxiety in dementia

Depression and anxiety are common emotional symptoms in patients with dementia. These symptoms can significantly impact quality of life for patients and caregivers, and can complicate the management of the disease. Below we will we will explore the relationship between depression and anxiety in dementia, including the challenges and considerations for healthcare providers.

Depression is common in patients with dementia and can manifest as a persistent feeling of sadness or hopelessness. Depression can exacerbate cognitive and behavioral symptoms of dementia, leading to decreased quality of life for patients and caregivers. Depression can also complicate the management of dementia by decreasing adherence to medication regimens and increasing the risk of adverse health outcomes. Management of depression in patients with dementia may include medication, psychotherapy, or behavioral interventions.

Anxiety is another common emotional symptom in patients with dementia. Anxiety can manifest as restlessness, agitation, or fear, and can significantly impact quality of life for patients with dementia. Anxiety can be caused by a variety of factors, including medication side effects, changes in the environment, or fear of the disease and its progression. Management of anxiety in patients with dementia may include medication, behavioral interventions, or modifications to the environment to promote feelings of safety and security.

It is important to note that depression and anxiety can also impact the progression of dementia. Patients with depression and anxiety may experience more rapid cognitive decline and increased risk of adverse health outcomes. Healthcare providers must consider the impact of depression and anxiety on the progression of dementia and work to manage emotional symptoms and promote positive mental health.

Additionally, the relationship between depression and anxiety in dementia is complex. Patients with depression may be more likely to experience anxiety, and patients with anxiety may be more likely to experience depression. Comorbid depression and anxiety can complicate the management of dementia, as both conditions must be managed simultaneously. Management of depression and anxiety in patients with dementia may require a combination of medication, psychotherapy, and behavioral interventions.

Finally, it is important to consider the impact of depression and anxiety on caregiver well-being. Caregivers of patients with dementia may experience increased stress and burden when managing emotional symptoms, leading to decreased quality of life and increased risk of burnout. It is important to provide caregivers with support and resources to manage the emotional needs of patients with dementia and to promote their own emotional well-being.

In conclusion, depression and anxiety are common emotional symptoms in patients with dementia that can significantly impact quality of life for patients and caregivers. Depression and anxiety can complicate the management of dementia and may require a combination of medication, psychotherapy, and behavioral interventions. Healthcare providers must consider the impact of depression and anxiety on the progression of dementia and work to manage emotional symptoms and promote positive mental health. Additionally, providing support and resources to caregivers is essential for managing the emotional needs of patients with dementia and promoting caregiver well-being.

Techniques for managing emotions

Managing emotions is an essential aspect of maintaining emotional well-being and mental health. This is particularly important in patients with dementia, who may experience emotional symptoms such as depression and anxiety. Below we will we will explore techniques for managing emotions in patients with dementia, including the challenges and considerations for healthcare providers.

One technique for managing emotions in patients with dementia is cognitive behavioral therapy (CBT). CBT is a psychotherapeutic approach that focuses on identifying and changing negative patterns of thought and behavior. CBT has been shown to be effective in managing depression and anxiety in patients with dementia. However, CBT may be challenging for patients with advanced dementia, who may have difficulty with memory and abstract thinking.

Another technique for managing emotions in patients with dementia is reminiscence therapy. Reminiscence therapy involves the use of memories and past experiences to promote emotional well-being. Reminiscence therapy can be effective in managing emotional symptoms such as depression and anxiety, as well as behavioral symptoms such as aggression and agitation. Reminiscence therapy may involve the use of photographs, music, or other sensory stimuli to evoke memories and promote emotional well-being.

Additionally, mindfulness-based interventions may be effective in managing emotional symptoms in patients with dementia. Mindfulness-based interventions involve the cultivation of present-moment awareness and non-judgmental acceptance of thoughts and emotions. Mindfulness-based interventions have been shown to be effective in managing depression and anxiety in older adults, including those with dementia. Mindfulness-based interventions may involve the use of meditation, breathing exercises, or other techniques to promote present-moment awareness and non-judgmental acceptance.

Another technique for managing emotions in patients with dementia is validation therapy. Validation therapy involves the validation of a patient's emotions and experiences, even if they are not factually accurate. Validation therapy can be effective in managing emotional symptoms such as anxiety and aggression, as it promotes feelings of safety and security in patients with dementia. Validation therapy may involve the use of empathy, validation, and redirection to manage emotional symptoms and promote positive emotional well-being.

Finally, it is important to consider the impact of the environment on emotional well-being in patients with dementia. Modifications to the environment, such as increased lighting or decreased noise levels, can promote feelings of safety and security and may reduce emotional symptoms such as anxiety and aggression. Additionally, providing activities and social engagement can promote positive emotional well-being in patients with dementia.

In conclusion, managing emotions is an essential aspect of maintaining emotional well-being and mental health in patients with dementia. Techniques for managing emotions in patients with dementia may include cognitive behavioral therapy, reminiscence therapy, mindfulness-based interventions, validation therapy, and modifications to the environment. Healthcare providers must consider the challenges and considerations for managing emotional symptoms in patients with dementia and work to promote positive emotional well-being. Additionally, providing support and resources to caregivers is essential for managing the emotional needs of patients with dementia and promoting caregiver well-being.

The role of therapy and counseling

Dementia is a progressive and debilitating condition that affects an individual's cognitive and emotional functioning. It is a chronic condition that requires long-term care and management, which can be challenging for both the patient and their caregivers. Therapy and counseling can play a crucial role in managing the emotional and behavioral symptoms of dementia, improving quality of life for the patient and their caregivers.

Therapy and counseling can help patients with dementia manage their emotional symptoms, such as depression, anxiety, and aggression. Patients with dementia may experience feelings of sadness, hopelessness, and loss of control, which can lead to depression. They may also experience feelings of fear, worry, and confusion, which can lead to anxiety. Therapy and counseling can help patients identify and express their emotions, develop coping strategies, and improve their overall emotional well-being.

Therapy and counseling can also help patients with dementia manage their behavioral symptoms, such as agitation, aggression, and wandering. These behaviors can be challenging for caregivers to manage and can impact the safety and well-being of both the patient and their caregivers. Therapy and counseling can help patients develop strategies for managing their behaviors, such as relaxation techniques, distraction techniques, and redirection.

There are several different types of therapy and counseling that can be effective in managing the emotional and behavioral symptoms of dementia. Cognitive-behavioral therapy (CBT) is a type of therapy that focuses on changing negative patterns of thought and behavior. CBT has been shown to be effective in managing depression and anxiety in patients with dementia. It can also be used to manage behavioral symptoms by helping patients identify and change negative thoughts and behaviors that contribute to their behaviors.

Reminiscence therapy is another type of therapy that can be effective in managing emotional symptoms in patients with dementia. Reminiscence therapy involves the use of memories and past experiences to promote emotional well-being. It can be effective in managing depression and anxiety by promoting feelings of safety and security in patients with dementia. Reminiscence therapy may involve the use of photographs, music, or other sensory stimuli to evoke memories and promote positive emotional well-being.

Validation therapy is another type of therapy that can be effective in managing emotional symptoms in patients with dementia. Validation therapy involves the validation of a patient's emotions and experiences, even if they are not factually accurate. Validation therapy can be effective in managing emotional symptoms such as anxiety and aggression, as it promotes feelings of safety and security in patients with dementia.

In addition to therapy and counseling for patients with dementia, it is important to provide support and resources for their caregivers. Caregivers of patients with dementia may experience feelings of stress, anxiety, and depression, which can impact their well-being and ability to provide care. Therapy and counseling can be effective in managing these emotional symptoms in caregivers, improving their overall well-being and ability to provide care.

In conclusion, therapy and counseling can play a crucial role in managing the emotional and behavioral symptoms of dementia, improving quality of life for the patient and their caregivers. Cognitive-behavioral therapy, reminiscence therapy, and validation therapy are effective types of therapy for managing emotional symptoms in patients with dementia. It is also important to provide support and resources for caregivers, including therapy and counseling to manage their emotional symptoms and improve their ability to provide care.

Chapter Nine

Caregiver Support

Dementia is a chronic condition that requires long-term care and management. Caregivers play a critical role in supporting individuals with dementia, providing assistance with daily activities and managing their emotional and behavioral symptoms. Caregiving can be challenging and stressful, and it is essential to provide support and resources for caregivers to promote their well-being and ability to provide care.

Caregivers of individuals with dementia may experience a range of emotional and physical symptoms, such as depression, anxiety, stress, fatigue, and social isolation. Caregiving can be a full-time job that requires significant physical and emotional energy, which can lead to burnout and caregiver fatigue. It is essential to provide caregivers with support and resources to manage their emotional and physical symptoms, promote their well-being, and improve their ability to provide care.

One way to provide support to caregivers is through caregiver education and training. Caregiver education programs can provide caregivers with the knowledge and skills they need to manage the daily care of individuals with dementia. These programs can include training on how to manage challenging behaviors, communication strategies, and how to provide personal care. Caregiver education can also provide information on community resources, such as support groups and respite care, to help caregivers manage their emotional and physical well-being.

Respite care is another way to support caregivers of individuals with dementia. Respite care provides temporary relief to caregivers by providing assistance with daily care and activities. This type of care can be provided in the home or in a residential care facility, allowing caregivers to take a break from their caregiving responsibilities and focus on their own well-being. Respite care can help prevent caregiver burnout and improve the overall quality of care provided to individuals with dementia.

Support groups are another valuable resource for caregivers of individuals with dementia. Support groups provide a safe and supportive environment for caregivers to connect with others who are going through similar experiences. Caregiver support groups can provide emotional support, practical advice, and information on community resources. They can also help caregivers develop coping strategies and manage their emotional well-being.

Technology can also be a valuable resource for caregivers of individuals with dementia. There are several technologies available that can assist with the care of individuals with dementia, such as GPS tracking devices, medication reminders, and communication devices. These technologies can help caregivers manage their daily care responsibilities, promote safety and independence for individuals with dementia, and reduce caregiver stress.

In addition to these resources, it is essential to provide caregivers with emotional support. Caregivers may experience feelings of guilt, grief, and loss as they navigate the challenges of caring for individuals with dementia. It is essential to provide caregivers with the opportunity to express their feelings, receive validation and support, and develop coping strategies to manage their emotional well-being.

In conclusion, caregiving for individuals with dementia can be challenging and stressful, and it is essential to provide caregivers with support and resources to manage their emotional and physical well-being. Caregiver education, respite care, support groups, technology, and emotional support are all valuable resources that can assist caregivers in their caregiving responsibilities. By providing caregivers with the support they need, we can improve the quality of care provided to individuals with dementia and promote the well-being of their caregivers.

Understanding the caregiver role

The caregiver role is an essential aspect of providing care to individuals with dementia. Caregivers play a critical role in managing daily activities, providing emotional support, and promoting the overall well-being of individuals with dementia. Caregiving can be a rewarding experience, but it can also be challenging and stressful. Understanding the caregiver role and providing support for caregivers is essential to ensure the well-being of both the caregiver and the individual with dementia.

The caregiver role involves managing daily activities, such as personal care, medication management, and household tasks. Caregivers may also need to manage challenging behaviors, such as aggression, agitation, and confusion. Caregivers must also communicate effectively with individuals with dementia, as communication difficulties are common in the later stages of the disease. Managing these responsibilities requires a significant amount of physical and emotional energy, which can lead to caregiver burnout and stress.

Caregiving can be emotionally challenging, as caregivers may experience a range of emotions, including grief, loss, guilt, and frustration. Caregivers may feel a sense of loss as they watch their loved one's cognitive abilities decline. They may also experience guilt if they feel they are not providing adequate care or if they need to seek outside help. It is essential to recognize and validate these emotions and provide emotional support to caregivers.

Providing support for caregivers is critical to ensure the well-being of both the caregiver and the individual with dementia. Caregivers can benefit from education and training programs that provide them with the knowledge and skills they need to manage daily care responsibilities effectively. These programs can include training on how to manage challenging behaviors, communication strategies, and personal care.

Respite care is another way to support caregivers. Respite care provides temporary relief to caregivers by providing assistance with daily care and activities. This type of care can be provided in the home or in a residential care facility, allowing caregivers to take a break from their caregiving responsibilities and focus on their own well-being. Respite care can help prevent caregiver burnout and improve the overall quality of care provided to individuals with dementia.

Support groups are also an essential resource for caregivers. Support groups provide a safe and supportive environment for caregivers to connect with others who are going through similar experiences. Caregiver support groups can provide emotional support, practical advice, and information on community resources. They can also help caregivers develop coping strategies and manage their emotional well-being.

Technology can also be a valuable resource for caregivers. There are several technologies available that can assist with the care of individuals with dementia, such as GPS tracking devices, medication reminders, and communication devices. These technologies can help caregivers manage their daily care responsibilities, promote safety and independence for individuals with dementia, and reduce caregiver stress.

In addition to these resources, it is essential to provide caregivers with emotional support. Caregivers may experience feelings of guilt, grief, and loss as they navigate the challenges of caring for individuals with dementia.

It is essential to provide caregivers with the opportunity to express their feelings, receive validation and support, and develop coping strategies to manage their emotional well-being.

It is also important to recognize the importance of self-care for caregivers. Caregiving can be a full-time job that requires significant physical and emotional energy. Caregivers must take care of themselves to ensure they are healthy and well-rested. This may include taking breaks, engaging in enjoyable activities, and seeking support from friends and family.

In conclusion, understanding the caregiver role and providing support for caregivers is critical to ensure the well-being of both the caregiver and the individual with dementia. Caregiving can be a rewarding experience, but it can also be challenging and stressful. By providing caregivers with education and training, respite care, support groups, technology, and emotional support, we can promote the overall well-being of individuals with dementia and their caregivers.

Managing caregiver stress and burnout

Caring for someone with dementia can be a rewarding experience, but it can also be stressful and emotionally challenging. Caregivers may experience feelings of burnout, exhaustion, and frustration as they navigate the challenges of caring for someone with dementia. It is essential to recognize and manage caregiver stress to ensure the well-being of both the caregiver and the individual with dementia.

Caregiver stress and burnout can manifest in several ways. Caregivers may experience physical symptoms such as fatigue, insomnia, and headaches. They may also experience emotional symptoms such as anxiety, depression, and irritability. Caregiver stress can affect overall health and well-being, making it essential to manage and reduce stress levels.

One way to manage caregiver stress is to practice self-care. Self-care includes taking care of physical and emotional needs, such as getting enough sleep, eating a healthy diet, engaging in regular exercise, and taking breaks when needed. Caregivers may also benefit from engaging in enjoyable activities, such as hobbies, socializing with friends and family, and practicing relaxation techniques such as meditation and deep breathing.

Another way to manage caregiver stress is to seek support from others. This may include joining a support group for caregivers, seeking counseling or therapy, or reaching out to friends and family for emotional support. Caregivers may also benefit from respite care, which provides temporary relief from caregiving responsibilities.

It is also essential to recognize and manage caregiver guilt. Caregivers may feel guilty for seeking outside help, taking a break from caregiving responsibilities, or experiencing negative emotions. It is important to recognize that these feelings are normal and valid and to seek support from others to manage them effectively.

Communication is also critical in managing caregiver stress. Caregivers may benefit from communicating openly and honestly with the individual with dementia and other family members involved in caregiving. Effective communication can help reduce misunderstandings, promote a sense of teamwork, and improve overall care.

It is also essential to set realistic expectations and goals for caregiving. Caregivers may feel a sense of pressure to provide perfect care for the individual with dementia. However, it is important to recognize that caregiving is a challenging role, and it is not always possible to provide perfect care. Setting realistic expectations and goals can help reduce stress and promote a sense of accomplishment.

In addition to these strategies, caregivers may benefit from seeking professional help. This may include seeking counseling or therapy from a mental health professional, seeking advice from a geriatric care manager or social worker, or consulting with a healthcare provider to manage symptoms of stress and burnout.

It is important to recognize that caregiver stress and burnout can have negative consequences for both the caregiver and the individual with dementia. Caregiver stress can lead to decreased overall well-being, increased risk of illness, and reduced quality of care provided to the individual with dementia. By recognizing and managing caregiver stress, caregivers can provide the best possible care to the individual with dementia while maintaining their own health and well-being.

In conclusion, managing caregiver stress and burnout is critical to ensure the well-being of both the caregiver and the individual with dementia. Caregiving can be a rewarding experience, but it can also be stressful and emotionally challenging. By practicing self-care, seeking support from others, managing caregiver guilt, setting realistic expectations, and seeking professional help when needed, caregivers can effectively manage stress and provide the best possible care to the individual with dementia.

Resources and support for caregivers

Caring for someone with dementia can be a challenging and rewarding experience. It can be emotionally and physically demanding, and caregivers may often feel overwhelmed or isolated. However, there are many resources and support available to help caregivers provide the best possible care for their loved ones.

One of the most important resources for caregivers of individuals with dementia is education. Understanding the disease and its symptoms can help caregivers better anticipate and manage challenges associated with caring for someone with dementia. Caregivers may benefit from attending workshops, seminars, or support groups that offer education on dementia and caregiving.

Another valuable resource is support groups. Support groups provide an opportunity for caregivers to connect with others who are experiencing similar challenges. Support groups may be available online or in-person, and they may be organized by community groups, advocacy organizations, or healthcare providers.

Respite care is another important resource for caregivers. Respite care provides temporary relief from caregiving responsibilities and allows caregivers to take a break and recharge. Respite care may be available through community organizations or healthcare providers.

In addition to respite care, caregivers may benefit from hiring in-home caregivers. In-home caregivers can provide additional support with tasks such as meal preparation, personal care, and medication management. In-home caregivers may be hired through a home care agency or privately.

Technology is also increasingly being used to support caregivers of individuals with dementia. Technology tools such as GPS tracking devices, medication reminders, and home monitoring systems can help caregivers manage caregiving responsibilities and ensure the safety of their loved ones.

Financial resources may also be available to help caregivers. Some states offer financial assistance for caregiving services through Medicaid or other programs. Additionally, veterans and their caregivers may be eligible for benefits through the Department of Veterans Affairs.

Caregivers may also benefit from consulting with a geriatric care manager. Geriatric care managers are professionals who specialize in coordinating care for older adults and their families. They can help caregivers navigate the healthcare system, coordinate care between different providers, and provide information on available resources and support.

Finally, it is important for caregivers to prioritize their own health and well-being. Caregivers may benefit from seeking counseling or therapy to manage the stress associated with caregiving. Exercise, healthy eating, and regular sleep are also important for maintaining overall health and well-being.

In conclusion, caring for someone with dementia can be challenging, but caregivers do not have to do it alone. There are many resources and support available to help caregivers provide the best possible care for their loved ones. Education, support groups, respite care, in-home caregivers, technology tools, financial assistance, geriatric care managers, and prioritizing self-care are all important resources that can help caregivers manage caregiving responsibilities and maintain their own health and well-being.

Chapter Ten

Legal and Financial Planning

Dementia is a progressive and debilitating disease that affects millions of individuals worldwide. In addition to the physical and emotional toll it takes on individuals and their caregivers, dementia can also have significant financial and legal implications. It is important for individuals and their families to plan ahead and make arrangements for managing their finances and legal affairs.

Legal planning is an important consideration for individuals with dementia and their families. Advance directives such as a living will and durable power of attorney for healthcare allow individuals to specify their wishes for medical treatment in the event that they become unable to communicate. Durable power of attorney for finances allows a trusted individual to manage an individual's financial affairs if they become incapacitated.

In addition to advance directives, estate planning is an important consideration for individuals with dementia and their families. Estate planning involves creating a will or trust that specifies how an individual's assets will be distributed after their death. It is important to consult with an attorney who specializes in elder law to ensure that legal documents are properly prepared and executed.

Financial planning is also an important consideration for individuals with dementia and their families. Individuals with dementia may require specialized care and may have medical and other expenses associated with their condition. It is important to plan ahead and consider options such as long-term care insurance, Medicaid, and other financial resources that may be available to help cover the costs of care.

It is important for individuals with dementia and their families to establish a system for managing finances. This may involve assigning a trusted family member or friend to handle financial affairs, or it may involve working with a financial advisor or accountant to establish a system for managing bills, expenses, and investments.

Social Security and other government benefits may also be available to individuals with dementia and their families. Individuals may be eligible for disability benefits, retirement benefits, and survivor benefits through Social Security. It is important to consult with a Social Security representative or financial advisor to determine eligibility and to ensure that benefits are properly managed.

Finally, it is important for individuals with dementia and their families to be vigilant against financial exploitation and scams. Individuals with dementia may be vulnerable to financial abuse, and it is important to establish safeguards such as monitoring financial accounts and limiting access to sensitive financial information.

In conclusion, legal and financial planning is an important consideration for individuals with dementia and their families. Advance directives, estate planning, and financial planning are all important components of a comprehensive plan for managing the financial and legal implications of dementia. It is important to consult with professionals who specialize in elder law and financial planning to ensure that legal documents are properly prepared and executed, and that financial resources are properly managed. Finally, it is important to establish safeguards to protect against financial exploitation and scams.

Advance directives and power of attorney

Advance directives and power of attorney are important legal documents for individuals to consider, especially for those with dementia. These documents provide guidance and instructions for medical and financial decisions in the event that an individual becomes incapacitated or unable to make decisions on their own.

An advance directive is a legal document that allows an individual to specify their wishes for medical treatment and end-of-life care. This document can include instructions for life-sustaining treatment, such as resuscitation or mechanical ventilation, as well as preferences for pain management and hospice care. Advance directives can help ensure that an individual's wishes are respected and followed, even if they are unable to communicate or make decisions for themselves.

1. A power of attorney is a legal document that designates a trusted individual to make decisions on an individual's behalf. There are two types of power of attorney: financial and healthcare. A financial power of attorney allows a designated individual to make decisions regarding an individual's finances, such as paying bills and managing investments. A healthcare power of attorney allows a designated individual to make medical decisions on an individual's behalf.

For individuals with dementia, advance directives and power of attorney can be especially important. Dementia is a progressive disease that can affect an individual's decision-making abilities, and it may eventually result in the individual being unable to make decisions for themselves. By creating advance directives and power of attorney early on, individuals with dementia can ensure that their wishes are respected and that their financial and medical affairs are managed according to their preferences.

It is important to note that advance directives and power of attorney must be created while an individual is still mentally competent and able to make decisions for themselves. Once an individual becomes incapacitated, it may be too late to create these documents. It is important to discuss these options with a trusted attorney or financial advisor to ensure that the appropriate legal documents are in place.

In addition to advance directives and power of attorney, there are other legal documents that individuals with dementia and their families should consider. These may include a living will, which specifies an individual's wishes for end-of-life care, and a revocable living trust, which allows an individual to transfer assets to a trust that is managed by a designated trustee.

Creating legal documents such as advance directives and power of attorney can be a difficult and emotional process. It is important for individuals with dementia and their families to discuss these options and make decisions together. It is also important to update these documents regularly to ensure that they reflect an individual's current wishes and circumstances.

In conclusion, advance directives and power of attorney are important legal documents for individuals with dementia to consider. These documents can help ensure that an individual's wishes for medical and financial decisions are respected and followed, even if they are unable to make decisions for themselves. It is important to discuss these options with a trusted attorney or financial advisor and to update these documents regularly to reflect an individual's current wishes and circumstances.

Long-term care planning and funding options

Long-term care planning and funding options are important considerations for individuals with dementia and their families. As dementia is a progressive disease, individuals with dementia often require long-term care services as their condition worsens. Long-term care can be expensive, so it is important to plan ahead and explore funding options to ensure that individuals with dementia can receive the care they need.

One option for long-term care funding is private insurance. Long-term care insurance can help cover the costs of care in a nursing home, assisted living facility, or in-home care services. It is important to purchase long-term care insurance early on, as premiums increase with age and health conditions. Some insurance policies may have restrictions on coverage for pre-existing conditions, including dementia, so it is important to carefully review policies before purchasing.

Medicaid is another funding option for long-term care. Medicaid is a government program that provides health insurance to low-income individuals and families. Medicaid covers long-term care services for individuals with limited income and resources. However, eligibility requirements vary by state, and not all long-term care services may be covered. It is important to research the eligibility requirements and coverage options in your state.

Veterans and their spouses may be eligible for long-term care benefits through the Department of Veterans Affairs (VA). The VA offers a range of long-term care services, including nursing home care, respite care, and in-home care. Eligibility requirements for VA long-term care benefits depend on the veteran's service history and disability status.

Another funding option for long-term care is personal savings and assets. Individuals with dementia and their families may choose to use personal savings or sell assets, such as a home or investments, to fund long-term care services. It is important to consult with a financial advisor to develop a plan for managing personal finances and assets to ensure that funds are available for long-term care.

In addition to long-term care funding options, it is important to consider long-term care planning. Long-term care planning involves identifying the types of care services needed and creating a plan for accessing those services. This may include creating a care team of healthcare providers and family members, developing a schedule for care services, and exploring options for in-home care, assisted living, or nursing home care.

It is also important to consider the individual's preferences for care, such as location, type of care, and cultural or religious considerations. Advance directives and power of attorney can help ensure that an individual's preferences for medical and financial decisions are respected and followed.

In conclusion, long-term care planning and funding options are important considerations for individuals with dementia and their families. Private insurance, Medicaid, VA benefits, personal savings and assets, and long-term care planning can all help cover the costs of long-term care services. It is important to research and explore these options early on and to consult with a financial advisor or attorney to develop a plan for managing finances and accessing care services. Long-term care planning can help ensure that individuals with dementia receive the care they need and that their preferences for care are respected and followed.

Navigating the legal and financial aspects of dementia care

Dementia is a complex and challenging condition that can have significant legal and financial implications for both individuals and their families. As the condition progresses, it can become increasingly difficult for individuals with dementia to manage their own affairs, including making decisions about their health care, finances, and living arrangements. It is important for individuals and families to plan ahead and make arrangements to ensure that they have the legal and financial support they need to manage the challenges of dementia.

One of the most important legal documents that individuals with dementia and their families should consider is a power of attorney. A power of attorney is a legal document that allows an individual to appoint someone else to make decisions on their behalf. This can include decisions about finances, property, and health care. A power of attorney can be particularly important for individuals with dementia, who may become unable to manage their own affairs as the condition progresses.

1. There are two types of power of attorney: a durable power of attorney and a springing power of attorney. A durable power of attorney remains in effect even if the individual becomes incapacitated, while a springing power of attorney only goes into effect if the individual becomes incapacitated. It is important to carefully consider the type of power of attorney that is appropriate for the individual's needs and circumstances.

Another important legal document that individuals and families should consider is an advance directive. An advance directive is a legal document that outlines an individual's wishes for medical care and treatment in the event that they become unable to communicate or make decisions for themselves. This can include decisions about life-sustaining treatment, such as feeding tubes and ventilators, as well as decisions about palliative care and end-of-life care.

In addition to legal planning, families also need to consider the financial implications of dementia care. Dementia can be a costly condition, with significant expenses associated with medical care, long-term care, and other support services. Families may need to explore a range of funding options to ensure that they have the resources they need to provide care for their loved one.

One potential source of funding for dementia care is long-term care insurance. Long-term care insurance can provide coverage for a range of services, including in-home care, assisted living, and nursing home care. It is important to carefully review the terms of the policy and consider factors such as premiums, deductibles, and coverage limits before purchasing long-term care insurance.

Another potential source of funding for dementia care is Medicaid. Medicaid is a joint federal-state program that provides health care coverage to individuals with low incomes and limited resources. Medicaid can cover a range of services, including long-term care, but eligibility requirements vary by state and can be complex. Families should consult with a Medicaid planning professional to determine if they are eligible for Medicaid and to explore their options for accessing benefits.

Finally, families may need to explore their options for paying for dementia care out of pocket. This can involve drawing on personal savings, selling assets, or exploring other funding sources. It is important to carefully consider the financial implications of each option and to consult with financial and legal professionals before making any decisions.

Navigating the legal and financial aspects of dementia care can be challenging and complex, but it is important for individuals and families to plan ahead and make arrangements to ensure that they have the support they need. By considering options such as power of attorney, advance directives, long-term care insurance, Medicaid, and personal savings, families can ensure that they are prepared to manage the challenges of dementia and provide the best possible care for their loved one.

Chapter Eleven

Dementia and Driving

Dementia is a debilitating condition that affects the cognitive and behavioral functions of the brain. It is a progressive disorder that primarily affects the elderly population, and it can cause significant challenges to daily living, including the ability to drive. Dementia can lead to impairment in critical areas such as judgment, attention, memory, and perception, which can make driving unsafe. Therefore, people with dementia must take measures to ensure their safety and that of other road users.

Driving is a complex activity that requires coordination between multiple cognitive functions such as perception, attention, and decision-making. Dementia can lead to a decline in these functions, making it challenging for individuals with the condition to operate a vehicle safely. In the early stages of dementia, some people may still have the ability to drive, but as the disease progresses, the risk of causing accidents on the road increases. Studies have shown that people with dementia are at higher risk of motor vehicle accidents than their healthy counterparts.

As dementia progresses, individuals may experience changes in their behavior and personality, including agitation, confusion, and anxiety, which can affect their ability to concentrate while driving. They may also experience physical changes such as decreased reaction time, vision problems, and difficulty with coordination. These changes can significantly impair driving performance, and as such, people with dementia must be evaluated to determine whether they can continue driving safely.

Healthcare providers play a critical role in assessing the driving abilities of people with dementia. They can evaluate the individual's cognitive and physical functions, including vision, coordination, and reaction time, to determine if it is safe for them to continue driving. Various tools and assessments can be used to evaluate driving fitness, including cognitive screening tests, on-road evaluations, and simulations.

In cases where it is determined that the individual is no longer fit to drive, it is important to ensure that they understand the reasons for this decision. Losing the ability to drive can be a significant loss for people with dementia, and it is essential to approach the situation with sensitivity and compassion. Caregivers and family members can help by providing alternative means of transportation, such as carpooling, public transportation, or hiring a driver.

It is crucial to involve family members and caregivers in the decision-making process about driving and dementia. They can help monitor the person's behavior and recognize changes that may impact driving safety. Family members and caregivers can also provide emotional support to the person with dementia during this challenging time.

In addition to healthcare providers, there are various resources available to individuals with dementia and their caregivers regarding driving safety. The Alzheimer's Association offers a guide for families and caregivers on driving and dementia, which includes information on warning signs, evaluation tools, and alternative transportation options. Additionally, some states have driver's license renewal requirements that include cognitive and physical evaluations for older adults, which can help ensure driving safety.

In conclusion, dementia can impact driving safety due to declines in cognitive and physical functions. Healthcare providers play a critical role in assessing driving fitness, and family members and caregivers can provide emotional support and alternative transportation options when driving is no longer safe. With proper evaluation and support, individuals with dementia can maintain their mobility and independence while ensuring the safety of themselves and others on the road.

Assessing driving ability

Assessing driving ability is an important consideration for individuals with dementia, as driving requires complex cognitive and physical abilities that can decline with the progression of the disease. Dementia can affect various cognitive functions such as memory, attention, perception, decision-making, and judgment, all of which are essential for safe driving.

The process of assessing driving ability in individuals with dementia can be challenging and requires a multidisciplinary approach involving healthcare professionals, family members, and sometimes, the department of motor vehicles (DMV). The assessment process typically involves several steps, including clinical evaluations, on-road driving evaluations, and communication with family members and caregivers.

Clinical evaluations are an essential part of the assessment process and can help healthcare professionals identify cognitive, visual, and motor impairments that may affect driving ability. The clinical evaluations may include cognitive tests, visual acuity tests, and motor assessments. These tests can help healthcare professionals identify deficits in areas such as memory, attention, perception, reaction time, visual acuity, and physical coordination.

In addition to clinical evaluations, on-road driving evaluations can provide valuable information about an individual's driving ability. On-road driving evaluations typically involve a driving instructor or occupational therapist accompanying the individual on a real-world driving test. During the test, the evaluator may observe the individual's ability to follow traffic laws, maintain proper speed, use turn signals, and navigate complex driving situations.

Communication with family members and caregivers is also an important part of the assessment process. Family members and caregivers can provide valuable information about an individual's driving behavior, such as difficulty with navigation, getting lost, or being involved in accidents. They may also be able to provide insight into the individual's overall cognitive and physical health, medication use, and any other factors that may affect driving ability.

If the assessment reveals that an individual's driving ability is impaired, it may be necessary to suspend or revoke their driving privileges. In some cases, the DMV may be involved in the decision-making process, especially if the individual is resistant to giving up their driving privileges. In these cases, the DMV may require a formal hearing to determine if the individual is fit to drive.

It is important to note that not all individuals with dementia will experience a decline in driving ability, and some may be able to continue driving safely for a period of time. However, as dementia progresses, the risk of accidents and injuries increases, and it is essential to monitor driving ability regularly.

In addition to assessing driving ability, there are steps that individuals with dementia and their caregivers can take to help maintain mobility and independence. For example, individuals with dementia can consider using public transportation, ride-sharing services, or community transportation programs. Caregivers can also help by providing transportation, scheduling appointments and outings during times when the individual is most alert and engaging in activities that promote physical activity and social interaction.

In conclusion, assessing driving ability is an important consideration for individuals with dementia. The process involves clinical evaluations, on-road driving evaluations, and communication with family members and caregivers. If driving ability is impaired, it may be necessary to suspend or revoke driving privileges. However, there are steps that individuals with dementia and their caregivers can take to maintain mobility and independence, such as using public transportation and engaging in physical activity and social interaction.

Strategies for discussing driving cessation

Dementia is a progressive neurological condition that affects memory, thinking, and behavior. As the disease progresses, individuals with dementia may experience a decline in their ability to perform everyday activities, including driving. This can be a challenging issue for caregivers and family members, as driving is often associated with independence and autonomy. However, it is important to prioritize safety for both the individual with dementia and others on the road. Below we will we will explore strategies for discussing driving cessation with someone with dementia.

Assessing driving ability is an important first step in determining whether or not someone with dementia should continue driving. Several tools are available to help assess driving ability in older adults, including those with dementia. These tools may include a driving evaluation by a trained professional or the use of standardized assessments such as the Clinical Dementia Rating Scale (CDR) or the Montreal Cognitive Assessment (MoCA). These assessments can help determine whether or not someone with dementia is able to safely operate a motor vehicle.

If an individual with dementia is deemed unfit to drive, it is important to discuss the issue with them in a sensitive and empathetic manner. Driving cessation can be a difficult topic to broach, as it may be seen as a loss of independence and control. It is important to approach the conversation with empathy and understanding, and to frame the issue in terms of safety rather than ability.

It is also important to involve the individual with dementia in the decision-making process as much as possible. This may include discussing alternative transportation options, such as public transit or ride-sharing services, or making arrangements for a friend or family member to provide transportation. It may also be helpful to involve the individual's healthcare provider in the discussion, as they can provide guidance and support for the transition to non-driving.

One effective strategy for discussing driving cessation with someone with dementia is to use "I" statements rather than "you" statements. For example, instead of saying "You shouldn't be driving," try saying "I'm concerned about your safety when you drive." This approach can help avoid placing blame on the individual and can create a more open and supportive dialogue.

It is also important to be prepared for resistance or denial from the individual with dementia. They may not fully understand the impact of their condition on their driving ability, or they may feel that they are capable of driving despite evidence to the contrary. In these cases, it may be helpful to involve a neutral third party, such as a healthcare provider or driving evaluator, to provide an objective assessment of their driving ability.

Another effective strategy is to frame driving cessation as a temporary measure. For example, you could suggest that they take a break from driving for a few weeks or months and then reassess their ability to drive at a later time.

This can help ease the transition and give the individual time to adjust to the idea of not driving.

It is important to remember that discussing driving cessation with someone with dementia is a difficult and emotional issue. It is important to approach the conversation with empathy, sensitivity, and understanding, and to involve the individual with dementia in the decision-making process as much as possible. With the right approach, it is possible to have a productive conversation about driving cessation that prioritizes safety and respects the individual's autonomy and independence.

Alternative transportation options

Dementia is a progressive condition that can affect a person's ability to perform daily activities, including driving. As the disease progresses, individuals with dementia may experience memory loss, confusion, and difficulty with decision-making, which can make driving unsafe. Therefore, it is important to consider alternative transportation options to ensure the safety of both the individual with dementia and others on the road.

There are several alternative transportation options for individuals with dementia, including public transportation, ride-sharing services, and specialized transportation services. Public transportation, such as buses and trains, can be an affordable and convenient option for those who are still able to navigate the system independently. However, it may be overwhelming for those with cognitive impairments or sensory issues, and may not be a practical option for those with mobility issues.

Ride-sharing services, such as Uber or Lyft, can be a convenient option for those who need door-to-door service and may be more comfortable with a familiar driver. These services can also be scheduled in advance, which can be helpful for those who may struggle with remembering appointments or schedules. However, individuals with dementia may become confused or disoriented during a ride, which could lead to safety concerns. Therefore, it is important to consider the level of cognitive impairment and overall safety when using ride-sharing services.

Specialized transportation services, such as medical transportation or non-emergency medical transport, can provide trained drivers and specialized vehicles equipped to assist individuals with dementia. These services can also provide door-to-door service and may be covered by insurance or Medicare. However, they may require advance scheduling and may have limited availability in some areas.

In addition to these transportation options, it is important to consider other strategies for managing transportation and mobility for individuals with dementia. For example, families and caregivers can consider reducing the need for transportation by providing opportunities for socialization and activities within the home or in a nearby community. Additionally, families and caregivers can work together to develop a transportation plan that addresses the individual's specific needs and limitations, such as identifying safe routes, scheduling appointments during times of day when the individual is most alert, and creating a visual schedule to help with reminders and planning.

It is important to note that giving up driving can be a difficult and emotional process for individuals with dementia and their families. However, it is important to prioritize safety and to consider alternative transportation options. Family members and caregivers can work together to provide emotional support and reassurance during this transition, and can also explore resources and support groups for individuals with dementia and their families.

In conclusion, managing transportation and mobility for individuals with dementia requires careful consideration and planning. Alternative transportation options, such as public transportation, ride-sharing services, and specialized transportation services, can provide safe and convenient options for those with dementia. Additionally, families and caregivers can work together to develop a transportation plan that addresses the individual's specific needs and limitations. By prioritizing safety and exploring alternative transportation options, individuals with dementia can continue to maintain their independence and participate in activities while also staying safe on the road.

Chapter Twelve

Dementia and Social Interaction

Dementia is a debilitating condition that affects cognitive abilities, including memory, language, and decision-making. As a result, individuals with dementia often experience challenges with social interaction, leading to feelings of isolation and loneliness. Below we will we will explore the impact of dementia on social interaction and provide strategies to support individuals with dementia in maintaining social connections.

The Impact of Dementia on Social Interaction

Dementia can impact social interaction in several ways. Firstly, individuals with dementia may experience difficulties with communication, including problems with language comprehension, word-finding difficulties, and reduced verbal output. This can make it challenging for individuals with dementia to express themselves and understand others, leading to social isolation and decreased participation in social activities.

Secondly, dementia can affect the ability to initiate social interactions, leading to reduced social participation. As dementia progresses, individuals may lose interest in previously enjoyed social activities or struggle to engage in new ones due to fear of failure or embarrassment.

Thirdly, behavioral and psychological symptoms of dementia (BPSD) can also impact social interaction. BPSD may include aggression, agitation, and apathy, leading to decreased engagement in social activities and withdrawal from social situations.

Strategies for Supporting Social Interaction

Despite the challenges of dementia on social interaction, there are several strategies that caregivers and loved ones can use to support individuals with dementia in maintaining social connections.

1. Adapt communication techniques: Communication can be enhanced by using simple, clear language, maintaining eye contact, and using non-verbal cues such as gestures and facial expressions. Using written cues, such as notes or pictures, can also aid communication and enhance social interaction.

2. Participate in structured activities: Structured activities can provide a sense of routine and purpose, helping individuals with dementia to remain engaged and connected. Activities can be tailored to individual preferences, such as music therapy, art therapy, or pet therapy.

3. Plan social outings: Outings with friends and family can be an excellent opportunity for social interaction. Planning activities that align with individual interests, such as visiting a favorite museum or park, can promote engagement and increase social connectedness.

4. Engage in reminiscence therapy: Reminiscence therapy involves discussing past experiences and memories. This can be a valuable tool for promoting social interaction and enhancing feelings of connectedness.

5. Create a dementia-friendly environment: Creating an environment that is welcoming and safe for individuals with dementia can help to reduce anxiety and promote social interaction. This may include minimizing distractions, providing clear directions, and using simple, recognizable signage.

6. Consider technology-based solutions: Technology-based solutions such as video calls, social media, and interactive games can provide opportuni-

ties for social interaction and engagement, even when in-person interaction is not possible.

Conclusion

Dementia can have a profound impact on social interaction, leading to feelings of isolation and loneliness. However, with appropriate support and intervention, individuals with dementia can continue to engage in social activities and maintain meaningful connections. Caregivers and loved ones can use a variety of strategies, including adapting communication techniques, participating in structured activities, and planning social outings, to promote social interaction and enhance the quality of life for individuals with dementia.

The importance of social connections

Dementia is a debilitating condition that can cause a range of cognitive, physical, and emotional symptoms. As the disease progresses, individuals with dementia may experience social isolation and withdrawal, which can negatively impact their overall well-being. Maintaining social connections is essential for individuals with dementia, as it can help them feel supported, engaged, and connected to their community.

One of the most common symptoms of dementia is memory loss, which can make it challenging for individuals to remember social connections and events. However, this does not mean that individuals with dementia cannot continue to enjoy social activities and interactions. In fact, research has shown that staying socially active can help slow the progression of dementia and improve quality of life.

Maintaining social connections can take many forms, including spending time with family and friends, participating in group activities, attending social events, and engaging in hobbies or other interests. For individuals with dementia, it may be helpful to focus on activities that are familiar and enjoyable, such as listening to music, playing games, or participating in art or dance classes.

It is also essential for caregivers and loved ones to support individuals with dementia in maintaining their social connections. This may involve scheduling regular visits or outings, arranging transportation to social events, and helping to facilitate meaningful interactions with others.

In addition to improving overall well-being, social connections can also have specific benefits for individuals with dementia. For example, engaging in social activities can help stimulate the brain and promote cognitive function. Social interaction has also been shown to reduce stress and anxiety and improve mood, which can be particularly beneficial for individuals with dementia who may experience emotional distress or agitation.

Overall, maintaining social connections is an essential aspect of dementia care. By staying socially engaged and connected, individuals with dementia can enjoy a higher quality of life and better overall health and well-being. Caregivers and loved ones can play a vital role in supporting individuals with dementia in maintaining their social connections and finding meaningful ways to engage with others.

Maintaining friendships and relationships

Maintaining friendships and relationships is an important aspect of life, and this is especially true for those who are living with dementia. Dementia is a condition that affects memory, thinking, and behavior, and it can cause individuals to withdraw from social interactions. However, it is important for those with dementia to maintain social connections as it can improve their quality of life and slow the progression of the disease.

One way to maintain friendships and relationships is through reminiscence therapy. This type of therapy encourages individuals with dementia to share memories of their past with their loved ones, which can help them to feel more connected and engaged in social interactions. Caregivers can also facilitate social activities such as group outings or game nights, which can provide opportunities for those with dementia to interact with others.

It is also important for caregivers to recognize that communication may become more difficult as the disease progresses. Individuals with dementia may have difficulty expressing themselves, understanding others, or recalling important details. Caregivers should be patient and understanding during interactions, and they should use clear and simple language when speaking with their loved ones. Nonverbal communication, such as gestures or facial expressions, can also be effective in communicating with those with dementia.

In addition to maintaining friendships and relationships with family members and friends, those with dementia can also benefit from forming new connections through support groups or day programs. These programs provide a safe and engaging environment for individuals with dementia to interact with others who are going through similar experiences. It can also provide a much-needed break for caregivers, who can feel overwhelmed by the demands of caring for someone with dementia.

Another way to maintain social connections is through technology. Social media platforms, video conferencing, and messaging apps can help individuals with dementia to stay connected with loved ones who may not be able to visit in person. This can be especially helpful for those who are living in care facilities or who have family members who live far away.

Maintaining friendships and relationships can also have physical benefits for those with dementia. Studies have shown that social interaction can improve cognitive function and reduce the risk of depression and anxiety. It can also improve overall physical health by reducing stress and increasing activity levels.

It is important for caregivers to be proactive in maintaining social connections for those with dementia. This can involve reaching out to family members and friends to schedule visits or engaging in social activities with their loved ones. Caregivers should also encourage their loved ones to participate in group activities or attend support groups.

In conclusion, maintaining friendships and relationships is crucial for individuals with dementia. Caregivers can facilitate social interactions through reminiscence therapy, social activities, and day programs. Clear and simple communication, as well as the use of technology, can also help individuals with dementia stay connected with their loved ones. Maintaining social connections can improve cognitive function, reduce the risk of depression and anxiety, and improve overall physical health.

Social activities and group programs

Social activities and group programs can play a vital role in improving the quality of life for people with dementia. Engaging in social activities can help individuals with dementia maintain a sense of purpose, reduce feelings of isolation and loneliness, and improve overall well-being. Furthermore, socialization can help individuals with dementia feel more supported, enhance their cognitive abilities, and increase their sense of independence.

There are many different types of social activities and group programs available for people with dementia. These can range from organized activities at senior centers and adult day care programs to informal social gatherings with family and friends. Some examples of social activities that have been found to be particularly beneficial for people with dementia include:

1. Music therapy: Music has been shown to have a powerful effect on individuals with dementia, and music therapy can be an effective way to improve mood, reduce anxiety, and increase social interaction.

2. Pet therapy: Animal-assisted therapy, or pet therapy, involves interaction with trained animals, such as dogs or cats, and has been found to reduce anxiety, depression, and loneliness in people with dementia.

3. Art therapy: Art therapy can be a way for individuals with dementia to express themselves creatively and engage in a meaningful activity that promotes social interaction.

4. Exercise programs: Exercise programs can help individuals with dementia maintain their physical health and mobility, while also providing opportunities for social interaction.

5. Support groups: Support groups can provide a safe and supportive environment for people with dementia and their caregivers to share experiences, offer emotional support, and learn from others in similar situations.

In addition to these specific programs, there are many ways that caregivers and family members can encourage social interaction for individuals with dementia. Some ideas include:

6. Encouraging participation in community events: Many communities offer events and activities specifically for older adults, such as senior centers or community centers.

7. Facilitating visits with family and friends: Maintaining connections with loved ones is important for socialization and emotional well-being.

8. Incorporating meaningful activities into daily routines: Engaging in activities that the person with dementia enjoys, such as gardening or cooking, can promote social interaction and provide a sense of purpose.

9. Creating a positive social environment: By creating a positive and supportive social environment, individuals with dementia are more likely to engage in social activities and maintain connections with others.

It's important to note that socialization for people with dementia may require some adaptations or modifications to accommodate changes in cognitive abilities or physical limitations. Caregivers and family members can work with healthcare professionals and social service providers to find appropriate activities and programs that meet the unique needs of the individual with dementia.

In conclusion, social activities and group programs can be a valuable tool in promoting social interaction and improving the quality of life for people with dementia. By offering opportunities for socialization, caregivers and family members can help individuals with dementia maintain a sense of purpose, reduce feelings of isolation, and improve overall well-being. Additionally, there are many different types of social activities and programs available, ranging from organized programs to informal social gatherings. By working with healthcare professionals and social service providers, caregivers and family members can find appropriate programs that meet the unique needs of the individual with dementia.

Chapter Thirteen

End-of-Life Care and Palliative Support

End-of-Life Care and Palliative Support

Dementia is a progressive condition that affects cognitive abilities, memory, and behavior. As the disease advances, individuals with dementia may experience increasing physical and emotional distress. End-of-life care and palliative support become essential to ensure comfort and dignity during the final stages of the disease. Below we will we will explore the various aspects of end-of-life care and palliative support for individuals with dementia.

End-of-Life Care

End-of-life care refers to the support provided to individuals in the final stages of life. It aims to ensure comfort and dignity during the end-of-life process. Individuals with dementia require specialized end-of-life care due to the unique challenges associated with the disease.

Symptom Management

Symptom management is a crucial aspect of end-of-life care for individuals with dementia. Pain, agitation, and other symptoms can cause significant distress in individuals with dementia, and it is essential to manage them effectively. Healthcare professionals may use medication or other non-pharmacological approaches to manage symptoms.

Advance Care Planning

Advance care planning involves making decisions about the care an individual would like to receive at the end of their life. It includes choosing a healthcare proxy, outlining treatment preferences, and discussing end-of-life care with loved ones. Advance care planning ensures that an individual's wishes are respected and that they receive care in line with their preferences.

Comfort Measures

Comfort measures aim to ensure that individuals with dementia are comfortable and free from pain and distress during the end-of-life process. It includes providing pain relief medication, hydration, and nutrition, and addressing other physical and emotional needs. Healthcare professionals may also use complementary therapies such as massage or music therapy to provide comfort.

Palliative Support

Palliative support aims to improve the quality of life for individuals with dementia and their families. It includes providing support and resources to manage symptoms, address emotional and spiritual needs, and prepare for end-of-life care.

Symptom Management

Symptom management is an essential component of palliative support for individuals with dementia. Healthcare professionals may use medication or other non-pharmacological approaches to manage symptoms such as pain, agitation, or sleep disturbances. Palliative support also includes addressing other physical symptoms, such as incontinence or difficulty swallowing.

Emotional Support

Dementia can cause significant emotional distress for individuals and their families. Palliative support includes addressing emotional needs, such as providing counseling or support groups for individuals and families. It also involves addressing spiritual needs, such as connecting with religious or spiritual communities.

Caregiver Support

Caregivers play a critical role in supporting individuals with dementia. Palliative support includes providing caregivers with resources and support to manage their own physical and emotional needs. It includes respite care, counseling, and other resources to help caregivers cope with the challenges of caregiving.

Hospice Care

Hospice care provides end-of-life care and support for individuals with a life-limiting illness, including dementia. Hospice care aims to ensure comfort and dignity during the end-of-life process. It includes symptom management, emotional and spiritual support, and caregiver support. Hospice care can be provided in the home or in a hospice facility.

Conclusion

End-of-life care and palliative support are crucial aspects of dementia care. It aims to ensure comfort and dignity during the end-of-life process and improve the quality of life for individuals with dementia and their families. Symptom management, advance care planning, comfort measures, emotional and caregiver support, and hospice care are all essential components of end-of-life care and palliative support for individuals with dementia. It is essential to address the unique challenges associated with dementia and provide specialized care to ensure that individuals with dementia receive the support they need to live comfortably and with dignity during the end-of-life process.

Hospice care for dementia patients

Dementia is a progressive disease that affects cognitive function, memory, behavior, and the ability to carry out activities of daily living. As the disease progresses, the need for specialized care becomes more evident. Hospice care is one form of specialized care that provides comfort and support for individuals with advanced dementia and their families. Below we will we will discuss hospice care for dementia patients, its benefits, and the eligibility criteria.

Hospice care is a type of care that focuses on improving the quality of life for people who have serious illnesses. Hospice care provides medical care, pain management, and emotional support to patients and their families. The goal of hospice care is to provide comfort and dignity to patients who have a life-limiting illness. Hospice care is provided by a team of healthcare professionals who are trained to care for people with serious illnesses.

Dementia is a chronic and progressive disease that can lead to a decline in cognitive function and physical health. Dementia patients often experience pain, confusion, and agitation in the later stages of the disease. Hospice care for dementia patients focuses on managing these symptoms and improving the patient's quality of life.

Hospice care for dementia patients can be provided in various settings, including the patient's home, a hospice facility, a nursing home, or a hospital. The care provided in hospice can include medical treatment, emotional support, and spiritual care. Hospice care for dementia patients can include the following services:

1. Pain management: Hospice care provides pain management services to help manage the physical pain and discomfort that patients may experience.

2. Personal care: Hospice care providers assist with personal care, such as bathing, dressing, and grooming.

3. Emotional support: Hospice care provides emotional support to both the patient and their family members. This can include counseling services and support groups.

4. Respite care: Hospice care providers can offer respite care to give family caregivers a break from their caregiving responsibilities.

5. Spiritual care: Hospice care providers can offer spiritual care to patients and their families, including religious services and support from a chaplain or spiritual advisor.

To be eligible for hospice care, patients must have a life expectancy of six months or less. However, dementia patients may be eligible for hospice care even if their life expectancy is longer than six months, as the disease can progress slowly over time. The eligibility criteria for hospice care for dementia patients include:

The patient has a diagnosis of dementia and has reached the advanced stages of the disease.

The patient has significant impairment in their activities of daily living, such as eating, dressing, and bathing.

The patient has frequent hospitalizations and emergency room visits.

The patient has a decline in their cognitive function and ability to communicate.

The patient has a decline in their physical health, such as weight loss or increased weakness.

Hospice care for dementia patients can provide many benefits. It can improve the quality of life for patients by managing their symptoms and providing emotional support. It can also reduce the burden on family caregivers by providing respite care and other support services. Hospice care can also help patients and their families prepare for end-of-life care and make decisions about advanced care planning.

In conclusion, hospice care is an important option for dementia patients and their families as the disease progresses to advanced stages. Hospice care can provide a range of services to manage symptoms, provide emotional support, and improve the patient's quality of life. To be eligible for hospice care, patients must meet specific criteria, including having a diagnosis of dementia and significant impairment in their activities of daily living. Hospice care for dementia patients can provide comfort and support to patients and their families during a challenging time.

Managing pain and comfort at end of life

Dementia is a progressive and ultimately terminal condition that affects a person's cognitive functioning, behavior, and physical abilities. As the disease progresses, individuals with dementia may experience pain and discomfort, which can be challenging to manage. It is crucial to provide end-of-life care and palliative support to individuals with dementia to ensure that they experience comfort and dignity in their final days.

Managing pain and comfort is a crucial aspect of end-of-life care for individuals with dementia. Pain and discomfort may be caused by a range of factors, including physical ailments such as infections, injuries, or chronic conditions like arthritis. However, individuals with dementia may also experience discomfort due to their cognitive and behavioral symptoms, such as anxiety, agitation, and depression.

Assessing and managing pain in individuals with dementia can be challenging due to their communication difficulties. Many individuals with dementia may not be able to express their pain verbally or may have difficulty identifying the location and intensity of their pain. Therefore, it is essential to observe nonverbal cues such as facial expressions, body language, and changes in behavior to identify signs of pain.

Nonpharmacological interventions can be effective in managing pain and discomfort in individuals with dementia. These include sensory interventions such as music, touch, and aromatherapy, which can help promote relaxation and reduce anxiety. Other interventions such as massage, heat and cold therapy, and gentle exercises like stretching can help alleviate pain and stiffness in the muscles and joints.

Pharmacological interventions may also be necessary to manage pain in individuals with dementia. However, care must be taken when prescribing medications, as individuals with dementia may be sensitive to the side effects of certain drugs. Pain medications such as acetaminophen and nonsteroidal anti-inflammatory drugs (NSAIDs) may be prescribed, but the dosage and frequency should be closely monitored.

Comfort care is also an essential aspect of end-of-life care for individuals with dementia. As the disease progresses, individuals with dementia may experience physical discomfort and decline, including loss of appetite, difficulty swallowing, and urinary incontinence. Comfort measures such as positioning, wound care, and hygiene can help promote comfort and prevent complications.

Hospice care is a specialized form of end-of-life care that focuses on providing comfort and dignity to individuals with terminal conditions, including dementia. Hospice care is typically provided in the home, nursing home, or hospice facility and involves a team of healthcare professionals who specialize in end-of-life care. The hospice team may include a physician, nurse, social worker, chaplain, and other professionals who work together to provide comprehensive care.

Hospice care for individuals with dementia may involve pain management, symptom relief, and emotional support for both the individual and their family members. The goal of hospice care is to ensure that the individual experiences comfort and dignity in their final days, and that their family members receive the support they need during this difficult time.

In addition to hospice care, palliative support can also be provided to individuals with dementia. Palliative care focuses on managing symptoms and providing emotional support to individuals with chronic conditions, including dementia. Palliative care can be provided in any setting and can be provided alongside curative treatments.

Palliative care for individuals with dementia may involve addressing symptoms such as pain, anxiety, and depression, as well as providing emotional and spiritual support to the individual and their family members. Palliative care can help individuals with dementia and their families cope with the challenges of the disease and provide comfort and dignity in their final days.

In conclusion, managing pain and comfort is a critical aspect of end-of-life care and palliative support for individuals with dementia. Care must be taken to identify signs of pain and discomfort and provide appropriate interventions, including nonpharmacological and pharmacological interventions.

Grief and bereavement support

Grief and bereavement are natural responses to losing a loved one, and these feelings can be especially difficult to navigate when caring for someone with dementia. As the disease progresses, caregivers may experience feelings of loss and grief as they watch their loved one's abilities decline. The death of someone with dementia can be especially complex, as it may feel like they have already been lost in some ways.

There are many ways that caregivers can cope with grief and bereavement while caring for someone with dementia. One important step is to acknowledge and accept the grief as a normal part of the caregiving experience. This can involve allowing oneself to feel and express emotions, such as sadness, anger, and frustration, in a healthy and constructive way. It can also involve seeking out support from others who have gone through similar experiences, whether through support groups or individual therapy.

It's important to remember that grief and bereavement don't end with the passing of a loved one. In fact, the process of grieving may continue long after the person with dementia has died. Caregivers may continue to experience feelings of sadness, guilt, and even relief as they adjust to life without their loved one.

One helpful strategy for coping with grief and bereavement is to focus on self-care. This can involve engaging in activities that bring joy and relaxation, such as exercise, hobbies, and spending time with friends and family. It can also involve seeking out professional help, such as therapy or counseling, to process emotions and develop coping strategies.

It's important for caregivers to recognize that grief and bereavement can also affect the person with dementia themselves, even if they may not be able to express it in the same way. Caregivers can help by providing comfort and support, such as through gentle touch and reassuring words. Hospice care can also be an important resource for managing end-of-life care and providing emotional support for both the person with dementia and their caregivers.

In addition to individual support, there are many resources available for caregivers who are coping with grief and bereavement. Support groups, both in-person and online, can provide a safe space for caregivers to connect with others who understand their experiences. Hospice and palliative care providers may also offer grief and bereavement services, including counseling and support groups.

It's important to remember that everyone grieves differently, and there is no "right" way to cope with the loss of a loved one. Caregivers may find that their feelings and experiences change over time, and that different strategies work best at different stages of the grieving process. By acknowledging and accepting grief as a natural part of the caregiving experience, caregivers can take important steps towards healing and finding support.

Chapter Fourteen

Dementia and the Arts

Dementia is a neurological condition that affects a person's memory, thinking, and behavior. It is a progressive disease that can cause significant cognitive decline and functional impairment. While there is no cure for dementia, there are several treatments and interventions available to help manage the symptoms and improve the quality of life of those affected by the disease. One such intervention that has gained popularity in recent years is the use of art and creative activities to engage individuals with dementia and support their well-being.

Art therapy is a form of therapy that involves using creative techniques such as painting, drawing, and sculpture to help individuals express themselves and communicate their feelings. It can be especially effective for people with dementia who may have difficulty communicating verbally. Art therapy can help people with dementia connect with others and express their emotions in a safe and supportive environment.

In addition to art therapy, there are several other ways that the arts can benefit people with dementia. Music therapy, for example, has been shown to improve mood, reduce anxiety, and improve overall quality of life for people with dementia. Singing, playing an instrument, or simply listening to music can help people with dementia connect with memories and emotions from their past.

Dance and movement therapies can also be beneficial for people with dementia. These therapies involve using movement to help improve balance, coordination, and mobility. They can also help reduce stress and anxiety and promote a sense of well-being.

One of the unique aspects of the arts is that they can be enjoyed and appreciated regardless of a person's cognitive abilities. Even individuals with severe dementia can still enjoy and benefit from creative activities. This is because art and creative activities can tap into a person's emotions and feelings, which are often still intact even when other cognitive abilities have declined.

The benefits of the arts for people with dementia are not just limited to the individual with the disease. Engaging in creative activities can also help caregivers and family members connect with their loved one and improve their relationship. Participating in art therapy or other creative activities together can create a positive and meaningful experience for both the person with dementia and their caregiver.

The arts can also provide a sense of purpose and meaning for people with dementia. Engaging in creative activities can give individuals a sense of accomplishment and a feeling of contributing to a larger community. It can help combat feelings of isolation and loneliness that are common among those with dementia.

There are several organizations and programs that are dedicated to promoting the use of the arts for people with dementia. The Alzheimer's Poetry Project, for example, is a program that uses poetry to help individuals with dementia connect with memories and emotions from their past. The program has been shown to improve mood, reduce anxiety, and increase social engagement among people with dementia.

The Museum of Modern Art in New York City offers a program called "Meet Me at MoMA," which provides guided tours and art-making activities for individuals with dementia and their caregivers. The program is designed to engage individuals with dementia in a meaningful and interactive way while also providing a supportive environment for caregivers.

In addition to these programs, there are also many resources available online for individuals and caregivers interested in using the arts as a form of therapy for dementia. The National Center for Creative Aging, for example, provides resources and information on the benefits of the arts for older adults, including those with dementia.

In conclusion, the arts can be a powerful tool for improving the quality of life for individuals with dementia. Art therapy, music therapy, dance and movement therapies, and other creative activities can help individuals with dementia connect with their emotions, improve their mood, and reduce feelings of isolation and loneliness. Engaging in creative activities can also provide a sense of purpose and meaning for people with dementia and their caregivers.

Art therapy for dementia patients

Art therapy has been shown to be an effective way to improve the quality of life for individuals with dementia. This approach to treatment uses art as a means of expression and communication, promoting emotional and cognitive well-being in patients. Dementia patients may experience a variety of symptoms such as anxiety, depression, agitation, and confusion, but art therapy has been found to help improve mood, increase communication, reduce stress, and enhance cognitive functioning.

Art therapy can take many forms, including painting, drawing, collage, and sculpture. The therapy sessions are usually led by a trained art therapist who provides guidance and support. The therapist may also use specific techniques such as guided imagery or mindfulness practices to help patients explore their emotions and experiences.

One of the benefits of art therapy for dementia patients is its non-verbal nature. Art can serve as a means of communication when verbal communication becomes difficult or impossible. Art therapists can help patients express their emotions, memories, and experiences in a safe and supportive environment. By providing a space for expression and communication, art therapy can help reduce feelings of isolation and loneliness that can be common among individuals with dementia.

Another benefit of art therapy is its potential to improve cognitive function in dementia patients. Research has shown that engaging in creative activities can help improve memory, attention, and other cognitive functions. This is particularly important for individuals with dementia, who may experience a decline in cognitive functioning over time. By engaging in art therapy, patients can stimulate their brain and improve their cognitive abilities.

In addition to improving cognitive function, art therapy can also help reduce agitation and anxiety in dementia patients. Art therapy provides a calming and relaxing environment, allowing patients to feel safe and secure. Patients may find that they are able to relax and let go of their worries, which can lead to a reduction in anxiety and agitation.

Art therapy can also be a valuable tool for caregivers and family members of individuals with dementia. Caregivers can participate in therapy sessions with their loved ones, providing an opportunity for shared experiences and memories. Caregivers may also find that they benefit from the therapy sessions themselves, as they are able to express their emotions and experiences in a safe and supportive environment.

Art therapy is a relatively low-risk treatment option for individuals with dementia. It does not involve the use of medications or invasive procedures, making it a safe option for many patients. It is also a non-invasive therapy, meaning that it does not require physical contact or invasive procedures. This can be particularly important for patients who are sensitive to touch or who have other physical limitations.

Overall, art therapy is a promising treatment option for individuals with dementia. It provides a safe and supportive environment for patients to express their emotions and experiences, and can help improve cognitive function, reduce agitation and anxiety, and improve overall quality of life. Art therapy can also provide a valuable tool for caregivers and family members, helping them to connect with their loved ones and find support during a difficult time.

Music and memory programs

Music has long been recognized as a powerful tool for emotional and psychological well-being, and its therapeutic effects are increasingly being recognized in the field of dementia care. Music can evoke memories, stimulate the brain, and provide a source of comfort and enjoyment for people with dementia. This has led to the development of music and memory programs, which have been shown to be effective in improving the quality of life for people with dementia.

Music and memory programs are based on the principle that music can access memories that are otherwise difficult to retrieve. This is because music is processed in multiple parts of the brain, including those involved in memory and emotion. Even in people with advanced dementia who have lost much of their ability to communicate, music can be used to access memories and stimulate cognitive function.

One of the most well-known music and memory programs is the Music & Memory program, which was developed by Dan Cohen, a social worker who recognized the power of music in dementia care. The program involves creating personalized playlists for each individual based on their musical preferences and life experiences. These playlists are then used to help stimulate memories and improve mood.

The Music & Memory program has been shown to have a number of benefits for people with dementia. One study found that after three months of participating in the program, participants had improved mood, increased socialization, and a reduction in the use of antipsychotic medications. Other studies have found that music can reduce agitation and improve sleep quality in people with dementia.

In addition to music and memory programs, music therapy is another approach that can be used to support people with dementia. Music therapy involves working with a trained music therapist to use music as a means of communication, expression, and emotional support. This can involve singing, playing instruments, or listening to music, and is tailored to each individual's needs and abilities.

Music therapy has been shown to be effective in reducing symptoms of depression, anxiety, and agitation in people with dementia. It can also help to improve communication, increase socialization, and enhance quality of life. One study found that music therapy improved overall well-being and cognitive function in people with dementia, as well as reducing behavioral and psychological symptoms.

In addition to music, other forms of art can also be used to support people with dementia. Art therapy, for example, involves using art as a means of communication, expression, and emotional support. This can involve drawing, painting, or other forms of artistic expression, and is tailored to each individual's needs and abilities.

Art therapy has been shown to be effective in reducing symptoms of depression and anxiety in people with dementia. It can also help to improve communication, increase socialization, and enhance quality of life. One study found that art therapy improved cognitive function and reduced agitation in people with dementia.

In conclusion, music and memory programs and art therapy are effective tools for supporting people with dementia. They can help to stimulate memories, improve mood, and reduce symptoms of depression, anxiety, and agitation. These approaches are tailored to each individual's needs and abilities, and can be used in a variety of settings, including care homes and community centers. With the growing recognition of the therapeutic effects of art and music, it is likely that these approaches will continue to be an important part of dementia care in the future.

Benefits of creative expression in dementia care

Creative expression has been found to have numerous benefits in dementia care. Dementia is a progressive cognitive decline that affects memory, language, and decision-making skills, among others. The condition is prevalent in older adults, and it is associated with a high burden of care for family and caregivers. Creative expression has become a popular intervention in dementia care due to its numerous benefits, including improving communication, reducing agitation and depression, and enhancing the overall quality of life.

Art therapy is one form of creative expression that has been found to be effective in dementia care. Art therapy involves the use of various art materials, such as paints, clay, and colored pencils, to help individuals express themselves creatively. It is a form of non-verbal communication that can help individuals with dementia who may have difficulty communicating verbally. Art therapy has been shown to reduce anxiety, depression, and stress in individuals with dementia.

Music therapy is another form of creative expression that has been found to be beneficial for individuals with dementia. Music has been found to activate multiple areas of the brain, including those involved in memory and emotion. Music therapy involves the use of music to help individuals with dementia recall memories, communicate, and engage with others. It has been found to improve mood, decrease agitation, and enhance overall quality of life in individuals with dementia.

Dance and movement therapy is another form of creative expression that has been found to be effective in dementia care. Dance therapy involves the use of movement to help individuals with dementia express themselves creatively. It has been found to improve mood, reduce agitation, and improve overall well-being in individuals with dementia. Dance therapy can also help improve physical functioning, balance, and coordination in individuals with dementia, which can help reduce falls and improve overall quality of life.

The benefits of creative expression in dementia care extend beyond the individual with dementia. Caregivers and family members can also benefit from participating in creative expression activities with their loved ones. Engaging in creative expression activities can help reduce stress, anxiety, and depression in caregivers and improve their overall well-being. It can also provide an opportunity for family members to connect with their loved one with dementia and improve their relationship.

In addition to improving mood and communication, creative expression has also been found to improve cognitive function in individuals with dementia. Studies have found that engaging in creative expression activities can help improve memory, attention, and executive function in individuals with dementia. This is likely due to the fact that creative expression activities engage multiple areas of the brain and require individuals to use a variety of cognitive skills.

Overall, the benefits of creative expression in dementia care are numerous. Engaging in creative expression activities can improve communication, reduce agitation and depression, enhance overall quality of life, and improve cognitive function. Caregivers and family members can also benefit from participating in these activities with their loved ones. Creative expression is a non-pharmacological intervention that can be easily incorporated into dementia care and has minimal side effects. As such, it is a valuable tool for improving the well-being of individuals with dementia and their caregivers.

Chapter Fifteen

Spirituality and Dementia

Dementia is a debilitating disease that affects millions of people worldwide. It can cause profound changes in behavior, personality, and cognitive function. In addition to the physical and mental challenges of dementia, it can also create a profound sense of loss and disconnection from the world. This is where spirituality comes in, as it provides a sense of purpose, meaning, and connection to something greater than oneself.

Spirituality is defined as a connection to a higher power, purpose, or meaning in life. It can include religious practices, belief systems, meditation, and other forms of personal reflection. Studies have shown that spirituality can have a positive impact on mental health, particularly in individuals with chronic illnesses or disabilities. In the case of dementia, spirituality can offer a sense of comfort, hope, and connection for both the individual with dementia and their loved ones.

One way that spirituality can be incorporated into dementia care is through religious practices. For individuals who have a religious affiliation, attending religious services, praying, or participating in religious activities can provide a sense of comfort and connection to their faith community. This can also be an opportunity for social interaction and support, as many religious organizations have support groups for individuals with dementia and their caregivers.

However, spirituality does not have to be limited to religious practices. Engaging in activities that bring a sense of joy and meaning, such as listening to music or spending time in nature, can also have a positive impact on an individual's mental and emotional well-being. Additionally, activities that encourage personal reflection, such as journaling or mindfulness meditation, can help individuals with dementia connect to a sense of purpose and meaning.

Spirituality can also be incorporated into dementia care through the use of spiritual care providers. These individuals are trained to provide spiritual support to individuals with dementia and their loved ones. They can offer spiritual guidance, facilitate spiritual activities, and help individuals explore their personal beliefs and values. Spiritual care providers can work in conjunction with healthcare professionals to provide holistic care to individuals with dementia.

It is important to note that spirituality is not a replacement for medical care or evidence-based interventions for dementia. Rather, it is a complementary approach that can provide additional support and comfort for individuals with dementia and their loved ones. It is also important to respect an individual's personal beliefs and values when incorporating spirituality into dementia care. For example, not all individuals with dementia may have a religious affiliation, and it is important to provide alternative forms of spiritual support that align with their personal beliefs and values.

In conclusion, dementia can be a challenging and isolating disease for both individuals with dementia and their loved ones. Incorporating spirituality into dementia care can provide a sense of comfort, connection, and meaning for those affected by the disease. Whether through religious practices, personal reflection, or the use of spiritual care providers, spirituality can be a valuable tool in dementia care. It is important to approach spirituality with respect for an individual's personal beliefs and values, and to incorporate it as a complementary approach to evidence-based interventions for dementia.

The role of faith and spiritual practices

Faith and spirituality play a significant role in the lives of many individuals, and this is no different for those living with dementia. While the cognitive and physical changes that occur with dementia can be distressing for the person affected, faith and spiritual practices can offer comfort and meaning in their lives.

For many people, their faith is an integral part of their identity, and dementia does not change that. However, the experience of dementia can raise complex questions about faith and spirituality, and caregivers must approach the topic sensitively.

The role of faith and spirituality in dementia care is multifaceted. For some people, it can provide a sense of comfort and peace during difficult times. For others, it may bring up feelings of confusion or frustration. Here are some ways in which faith and spirituality can impact the lives of those living with dementia:

Coping with Loss

Faith can provide a sense of comfort and peace to individuals with dementia as they navigate the many losses associated with the disease. As dementia progresses, people may experience the loss of their memories, independence, and sense of self. Faith can help individuals come to terms with these losses and provide hope for the future.

Providing a Sense of Purpose

Spirituality and faith can also provide a sense of purpose and meaning for individuals with dementia. They may find comfort in knowing that their life has a higher purpose and that they are part of something larger than themselves. This can help individuals maintain a sense of dignity and value, even as their cognitive and physical abilities decline.

Connecting with Others

Faith and spirituality can also provide opportunities for individuals with dementia to connect with others who share similar beliefs and values. This can be especially important for those who may have lost social connections due to the disease. Participation in religious or spiritual activities can provide a sense of belonging and social support, which can improve overall well-being.

Addressing End-of-Life Issues

Faith and spirituality can also play a significant role in end-of-life care for individuals with dementia. Many religious traditions have specific practices or rituals that can provide comfort and meaning for the dying and their loved ones. Faith can provide a framework for addressing difficult end-of-life issues, such as forgiveness, letting go, and finding peace.

Caregivers can support the spiritual and religious needs of those with dementia by being sensitive and respectful of their beliefs. This may involve providing opportunities for individuals to participate in religious or spiritual activities, providing access to religious leaders, or simply listening to their spiritual concerns.

It is important to note that the role of faith and spirituality in dementia care can be complex and varies from person to person. Some individuals may find comfort in their faith, while others may struggle with feelings of doubt or anger. Caregivers must approach the topic with sensitivity and respect for each person's unique beliefs and experiences.

In conclusion, faith and spirituality can play an essential role in the lives of individuals living with dementia. It can provide comfort, meaning, and a sense of purpose during difficult times. Caregivers must be sensitive and respectful of each person's beliefs, and provide opportunities for them to connect with others who share similar beliefs and values. By doing so, individuals with dementia can maintain a sense of dignity, value, and purpose, even as the disease progresses.

Religious and spiritual support for individuals with dementia

Religious and spiritual beliefs can be a source of comfort and support for individuals with dementia, their families, and caregivers. As a progressive disease, dementia can be challenging and isolating, but religious and spiritual practices can provide a sense of meaning and purpose, as well as a feeling of connectedness to something larger than oneself.

For many individuals with dementia, their religious or spiritual beliefs are an integral part of their identity and have been a source of comfort and guidance throughout their lives. These beliefs may continue to be important to them as they navigate the challenges of dementia, providing a sense of continuity and stability in the face of a changing reality.

Research has shown that engagement in religious and spiritual activities can have positive effects on the mental and physical health of individuals with dementia. Studies have found that participation in religious or spiritual activities can decrease symptoms of depression, anxiety, and agitation, while increasing feelings of well-being and quality of life. Additionally, religious and spiritual practices can provide a sense of community and social support, which can be especially important for individuals with dementia who may be at risk of social isolation.

Faith-based organizations can also provide valuable resources and support for individuals with dementia and their families. Many religious organizations offer support groups, counseling services, and other programs that can help individuals with dementia and their loved ones cope with the challenges of the disease. These programs can also provide opportunities for individuals with dementia to remain engaged in their faith communities and to continue to participate in activities that are meaningful to them.

In addition to formal religious or spiritual practices, there are many ways that caregivers and loved ones can support the spiritual well-being of individuals with dementia. This may include reading from religious texts, playing music or hymns, or simply engaging in activities that bring the individual a sense of comfort or joy.

It is important to note that spirituality and religion are deeply personal and individual experiences, and that individuals with dementia may have different needs and preferences when it comes to spiritual support. Some individuals may find comfort in traditional religious practices, while others may prefer more informal or personal expressions of spirituality. Caregivers and loved ones should be sensitive to the individual needs and preferences of the person with dementia, and should work to create an environment that is supportive and respectful of their spiritual beliefs.

It is also important to recognize that individuals with dementia may experience changes in their religious or spiritual beliefs as the disease progresses. For some, this may involve a shift away from formal religious practices or a re-examination of their beliefs. Caregivers and loved ones should be open to these changes and should support the individual in their exploration of their spirituality and faith.

In conclusion, religious and spiritual practices can provide a source of comfort, meaning, and connection for individuals with dementia, their families, and caregivers. Engagement in spiritual practices has been shown to have positive effects on the mental and physical health of individuals with dementia, and can help to foster a sense of community and social support. Caregivers and loved ones should be sensitive to the individual needs and preferences of the person with dementia, and should work to create an environment that is supportive and respectful of their spiritual beliefs.

Spiritual care at the end of life

Dementia is a progressive and debilitating disease that affects millions of people around the world. As the disease progresses, individuals with dementia may experience significant physical, cognitive, and emotional changes that can impact their sense of self and their relationships with others. In addition to medical and psychological interventions, many people with dementia and their families turn to spiritual care as a means of finding comfort, meaning, and hope during this difficult time.

Spirituality can be broadly defined as a person's search for meaning, purpose, and connection to something greater than themselves. For many people, spirituality is closely tied to religious beliefs and practices, while for others, it may be more of a general sense of connection to nature, community, or humanity. Regardless of one's specific beliefs, spirituality can be a source of strength and comfort during times of illness, loss, and transition.

For individuals with dementia, spiritual care can take many different forms. For those who have a religious affiliation, spiritual care may involve visits from a clergy member, participation in religious services or rituals, or prayer and meditation. For others, spiritual care may involve spending time in nature, listening to music or engaging in other creative pursuits, or connecting with others who share similar experiences or values.

One of the benefits of spiritual care is that it can help individuals with dementia feel a sense of connection and belonging, even as their cognitive and physical abilities decline. Spirituality can provide a sense of purpose and meaning, which can be especially important for individuals who may feel disconnected from their previous identities or roles as their disease progresses. Additionally, spiritual care can help individuals and their families cope with the grief and loss that often accompany dementia, as well as the uncertainty and anxiety about the future.

There are many different ways that caregivers and healthcare providers can incorporate spiritual care into dementia care. For example, staff at long-term care facilities can make sure that residents have access to religious services, spiritual reading materials, or other resources that may be meaningful to them. Family members can help their loved ones with dementia by providing opportunities for prayer, meditation, or other spiritual practices that align with their loved one's beliefs and values. Healthcare providers can also be trained to provide spiritual care, including active listening, presence, and empathy, as well as referral to spiritual or religious leaders when appropriate.

End-of-life care is a particularly important time for spiritual care for individuals with dementia. Many people turn to spirituality or religion as a means of finding comfort and solace during the dying process. Hospice and palliative care providers can offer a variety of spiritual care interventions, including chaplaincy services, music therapy, and support groups, to help individuals and their families navigate this difficult time. Spiritual care can help individuals with dementia find peace and meaning in their final days, and can provide families with a sense of comfort and support as they grieve.

It's important to note that not everyone with dementia may be interested in or benefit from spiritual care. Additionally, it's important to respect individuals' religious and spiritual beliefs and practices, and to avoid imposing one's own beliefs on others. When incorporating spiritual care into dementia care, it's important to approach each individual with openness and respect, and to tailor spiritual interventions to meet their unique needs and preferences.

In conclusion, spiritual care can be a valuable and meaningful aspect of dementia care. By addressing the spiritual needs of individuals with dementia and their families, caregivers and healthcare providers can help promote a sense of connection, meaning, and purpose, even as the disease progresses. Whether through religious practices, creative expression, or other means, spiritual care can help individuals with dementia find comfort, solace, and hope during this challenging time.

Chapter Sixteen

Dementia-Friendly Communities

Dementia is a chronic and progressive disease that can greatly affect the lives of individuals and their families. As the population ages, the number of individuals living with dementia is increasing, making it essential to create dementia-friendly communities. These communities are designed to create an environment that supports and engages individuals with dementia, while also educating the broader community about the disease.

A dementia-friendly community is a place where people living with dementia are respected, understood, and supported. This includes the physical environment, as well as the attitudes and behaviors of those living in the community. Dementia-friendly communities promote social inclusion and ensure that individuals with dementia are able to participate fully in community life.

One important aspect of dementia-friendly communities is the physical environment. This can include simple changes, such as signage that is easy to read and understand, or more significant changes, such as modifications to public buildings and transportation to make them more accessible to those with dementia. For example, creating clear pathways and reducing clutter can help reduce confusion and anxiety in individuals with dementia. Adding handrails and non-slip surfaces can also help prevent falls, which is a major concern for those with dementia.

Another important aspect of dementia-friendly communities is education and awareness. The community should be educated on the signs and symptoms of dementia, as well as how to interact with individuals who have the disease. This can include training for business owners and employees, community groups, and local law enforcement. Raising awareness about dementia can also help reduce stigma and encourage individuals to seek early diagnosis and treatment.

Dementia-friendly communities also prioritize social inclusion. This can include activities and programs that are specifically designed for individuals with dementia, as well as opportunities for those with dementia to participate in existing community programs. For example, some communities have created dementia-friendly choirs, where individuals with dementia can sing and perform together. Other communities have created memory cafes, which are social gatherings where individuals with dementia and their caregivers can meet and socialize in a supportive environment.

There are several benefits to creating dementia-friendly communities. One of the main benefits is that it can help individuals with dementia maintain their independence and quality of life. Dementia-friendly communities can also help reduce the burden on caregivers by providing additional support and resources. In addition, creating dementia-friendly communities can have a positive impact on the broader community by increasing awareness and understanding of dementia.

Creating dementia-friendly communities requires collaboration and support from community members, businesses, and local government. It is important to involve individuals with dementia and their caregivers in the planning process to ensure that their needs are being met. Funding and resources may also be necessary to implement changes to the physical environment and create programs and activities for individuals with dementia.

In conclusion, dementia-friendly communities are essential to support individuals with dementia and their families. These communities prioritize accessibility, education, and social inclusion to create an environment that supports and engages individuals with dementia. Creating dementia-friendly communities requires collaboration and support from community members and local government, but the benefits can be significant for individuals with dementia and the broader community.

Creating supportive environments

Dementia is a debilitating condition that affects millions of people worldwide. As the population ages, the number of people living with dementia is expected to increase significantly. The condition can cause significant challenges in daily life, including memory loss, confusion, and difficulty with communication. Creating supportive environments can help individuals with dementia lead better lives by providing them with a sense of safety and familiarity.

Creating a supportive environment involves adapting the physical and social environments to accommodate the unique needs of individuals with dementia. Some of the strategies that can be employed to create a supportive environment include modifying the home environment, providing appropriate lighting and visual cues, and fostering social connections.

Modifying the home environment is an important consideration for individuals with dementia. It is important to create a space that is safe and secure, yet also allows for independence and autonomy. This may involve making changes to the physical environment, such as removing clutter, creating clear pathways, and installing grab bars and handrails. It may also involve providing specialized equipment, such as walkers or wheelchairs, to help with mobility.

Providing appropriate lighting and visual cues can also help individuals with dementia feel more comfortable in their environment. Bright lighting can help to reduce confusion and disorientation, while color-coded labels and signs can help to make it easier to navigate the space. It is also important to minimize noise and distractions, as these can be overwhelming for individuals with dementia.

Fostering social connections is another important aspect of creating a supportive environment for individuals with dementia. Social isolation can exacerbate the symptoms of dementia, so it is important to create opportunities for social interaction and engagement. This may involve organizing social activities, such as games or outings, or simply spending time with friends and family.

In addition to modifying the physical and social environments, it is important to provide appropriate support and care for individuals with dementia. This may involve providing specialized care, such as medication management or assistance with daily tasks, as well as emotional support and counseling. Caregivers and family members can also benefit from support and education, as caring for someone with dementia can be challenging and overwhelming.

Creating a supportive environment can have a significant impact on the lives of individuals with dementia. By adapting the physical and social environments to accommodate their unique needs, individuals with dementia can maintain a sense of independence and dignity. This can lead to improved quality of life and overall well-being.

In conclusion, creating a supportive environment is essential for individuals with dementia. It involves modifying the physical and social environments to accommodate their unique needs and providing appropriate support and care. By fostering social connections, providing appropriate lighting and visual cues, and modifying the home environment, individuals with dementia can lead better lives and maintain a sense of independence and autonomy. Caregivers and family members can also benefit from education and support, as caring for someone with dementia can be challenging and overwhelming. Creating a dementia-friendly community requires a collective effort to make our communities safe, supportive, and inclusive for people with dementia.

Public awareness and education initiatives

Public awareness and education initiatives are critical in addressing the challenges associated with dementia. Dementia is a progressive and incurable disease that affects cognitive and functional abilities. It is a growing global public health concern, with an estimated 50 million people living with the condition worldwide, and this number is expected to triple by 2050.

Dementia is a complex and challenging disease that affects individuals, families, and communities. It is often associated with stigma, misunderstanding, and isolation. Public awareness and education initiatives play an essential role in reducing the stigma, increasing understanding, and improving support for people with dementia and their families.

One key initiative in raising public awareness and education on dementia is the World Alzheimer's Month. It is an international campaign that takes place every September, aimed at raising awareness and challenging the stigma surrounding dementia. It encourages individuals, organizations, and governments to take action and support those affected by the condition. World Alzheimer's Month provides an opportunity to raise awareness of the challenges of living with dementia and the importance of early diagnosis, access to support, and quality care.

Education initiatives are also critical in providing accurate and up-to-date information about dementia. Programs that target healthcare professionals, social workers, caregivers, and the general public can help increase knowledge and understanding of the condition. These programs can cover topics such as early detection and diagnosis, communication strategies, managing behavioral and psychological symptoms, and providing person-centered care.

Public awareness and education initiatives can also help to promote dementia-friendly communities. These communities are designed to create a supportive environment for people with dementia and their families. They aim to raise awareness, reduce stigma, and provide practical support to enable people with dementia to live as independently as possible.

Dementia-friendly communities can take various forms, from physical changes to the environment to the promotion of inclusive practices. Examples of physical changes include providing clear signage, reducing noise levels, and designing buildings that are dementia-friendly. Inclusive practices can include training staff to communicate effectively with people with dementia, promoting social activities, and providing education and support for caregivers.

Public awareness and education initiatives also play a crucial role in promoting research into the causes and treatments for dementia. Increased public awareness can help to increase funding for research and encourage participation in clinical trials. This can lead to improved understanding of the condition and the development of new treatments that can slow down its progression or provide relief from symptoms.

In conclusion, public awareness and education initiatives are critical in addressing the challenges associated with dementia. They play an essential role in reducing stigma, increasing understanding, and improving support for people with dementia and their families. Initiatives such as World Alzheimer's Month, education programs, and dementia-friendly communities are all examples of ways that public awareness and education can make a significant impact. By promoting research, increasing funding, and encouraging participation in clinical trials, these initiatives can help to improve the lives of people living with dementia and their families.

Community resources and support

Dementia is a progressive disease that can be emotionally, physically, and financially challenging for both patients and their families. In addition to medical care, there are many community resources and support options available to help individuals with dementia and their caregivers. These resources can provide a range of services, from information and education to support groups and respite care.

One valuable resource is the Alzheimer's Association, which provides information, education, and support for individuals with dementia and their families. The organization offers support groups, educational seminars, and a 24/7 helpline that provides information and support to anyone affected by dementia. The Alzheimer's Association also provides a range of online resources, including information about the disease, caregiving tips, and resources for finding local services.

Another resource is the National Institute on Aging, which provides information on dementia and resources for caregivers. The institute offers tips for communicating with individuals with dementia, strategies for managing behavior changes, and information about legal and financial planning. The National Institute on Aging also provides a range of online resources, including fact sheets and educational videos.

Local community resources can also be valuable for individuals with dementia and their families. Many cities and towns offer support groups for individuals with dementia and their caregivers. These groups can provide emotional support, as well as practical advice for managing the challenges of caregiving. Some communities also offer respite care, which provides temporary relief for caregivers so that they can take a break from their caregiving responsibilities.

Senior centers are another valuable resource for individuals with dementia and their families. Senior centers often offer a range of programs and services, including exercise classes, educational seminars, and social activities. Many senior centers also offer support groups for individuals with dementia and their caregivers.

In addition to community resources, there are also a variety of private organizations that offer support for individuals with dementia and their families. These organizations can provide a range of services, from medical care to in-home assistance. Some organizations also provide financial assistance for individuals who cannot afford medical care or other services.

It is important for individuals with dementia and their families to take advantage of the resources available to them. These resources can help provide emotional support, practical advice, and valuable services that can make life with dementia more manageable. By staying informed and connected to the community, individuals with dementia and their families can better navigate the challenges of the disease and maintain their quality of life.

Chapter Seventeen

Dementia and Cultural Diversity

Dementia is a progressive neurological condition that affects a person's cognitive abilities, including memory, thinking, and communication. It can impact people from all walks of life, regardless of age, gender, or ethnicity. However, cultural diversity and ethnicity can play a significant role in how dementia is experienced and perceived. Below we will we will explore the unique challenges that people from diverse cultural backgrounds face when it comes to dementia care.

Cultural diversity can impact every aspect of dementia care, from diagnosis to end-of-life care. Misconceptions and stigmas about dementia can be prevalent in some cultures, which can cause people to delay seeking medical help or to reject a diagnosis altogether. In some cultures, dementia is seen as a natural part of aging or a spiritual affliction, rather than a medical condition that requires professional intervention. As a result, people with dementia from these cultures may be reluctant to take medication or participate in traditional treatments.

Furthermore, the way people with dementia express their symptoms and emotions can also vary depending on their cultural background. For example, people from collectivist cultures may express their distress in more subtle and indirect ways, whereas people from individualistic cultures may be more likely to vocalize their distress. Therefore, healthcare professionals need to understand how cultural background can affect communication and be mindful of cultural differences when assessing and treating people with dementia.

Cultural background can also impact the type of care and support that people with dementia receive. For example, some cultures place a high value on family caregiving and may resist placing their loved ones in residential care facilities. Others may not have the same support systems in place, making it challenging to provide adequate care for someone with dementia at home. Healthcare professionals need to be aware of these cultural differences and work collaboratively with families to provide culturally sensitive care that meets the unique needs of the individual.

Another challenge facing people with dementia from diverse cultural backgrounds is access to appropriate care and support services. Cultural barriers such as language and limited understanding of available services can create significant obstacles for people from non-English-speaking backgrounds. In addition, some cultures may have different expectations and beliefs about the role of healthcare professionals, which can impact their willingness to engage with formal services.

To overcome these barriers, healthcare providers need to work closely with families and community organizations to create culturally responsive care plans. This might involve hiring bilingual staff or providing translated materials, offering culturally appropriate activities and programs, and developing relationships with community leaders to promote dementia awareness.

Despite these challenges, there are many examples of successful dementia care initiatives that have been tailored to meet the needs of people from diverse cultural backgrounds. For example, the Chinese Alzheimer's Society in Canada offers programs that cater to the unique needs of Chinese families, including language-specific support groups, educational workshops, and cultural activities. In Australia, the Italian-speaking Dementia Support Group provides a culturally appropriate environment for Italian-speaking people with dementia and their families to receive information, support, and socialization.

In conclusion, dementia is a complex condition that affects people from all cultures and backgrounds. Healthcare providers must recognize the unique challenges faced by people with dementia from diverse cultural backgrounds and provide culturally sensitive care that meets their individual needs. By working collaboratively with families and community organizations, healthcare providers can create supportive environments that promote the well-being and dignity of people with dementia, regardless of their cultural background.

Cultural considerations in dementia care

Dementia is a global health issue that affects individuals from all walks of life and cultures. It is a condition that affects memory, thinking, behavior, and the ability to perform daily activities. While the symptoms of dementia are universal, cultural factors play an important role in the way the condition is perceived, diagnosed, and treated. Therefore, it is essential for healthcare professionals to consider cultural factors when providing care for individuals with dementia.

The first step in providing culturally competent care for individuals with dementia is to understand how cultural values, beliefs, and practices may impact the individual's experience with the condition. For example, in some cultures, memory loss may be seen as a natural part of aging or a result of spiritual causes, rather than a medical condition. This may impact an individual's willingness to seek medical help for their symptoms. It is also important to consider how cultural norms and expectations may impact the family's experience of caring for a loved one with dementia. In some cultures, it is expected that family members will provide all of the care for their loved ones, while in others, it may be more common to rely on professional caregivers or community resources.

In addition to cultural considerations, it is important for healthcare professionals to have an understanding of the individual's background and personal history. This includes their education level, occupation, and socioeconomic status. These factors may impact the individual's ability to access healthcare resources or understand their diagnosis and treatment options. It may also impact their willingness to disclose their symptoms or seek help.

One approach to providing culturally competent care for individuals with dementia is to use a person-centered approach. This means that healthcare professionals should focus on the individual's unique needs, preferences, and experiences. This may involve working with family members or caregivers to understand the individual's cultural background and personal history. It may also involve adapting care plans to meet the individual's needs and preferences, such as incorporating cultural traditions or practices into daily activities.

Another important aspect of culturally competent care for individuals with dementia is to provide education and support to families and caregivers. This may involve providing information about the condition, treatment options, and community resources. It may also involve providing support and counseling to help families cope with the emotional and practical challenges of caring for a loved one with dementia. Healthcare professionals should also be aware of cultural differences in communication styles and use culturally appropriate communication techniques to help families and caregivers understand and manage the condition.

Community resources and support are also important for individuals with dementia and their families. In some cultures, there may be a stigma associated with dementia or mental illness, which may prevent individuals from seeking help or participating in community activities. Healthcare professionals can help to reduce this stigma by raising awareness about the condition and providing education to the community. They can also work with community leaders and organizations to create dementia-friendly environments and support groups for individuals and families affected by the condition.

In conclusion, providing culturally competent care for individuals with dementia is essential for improving outcomes and quality of life. Healthcare professionals should take into account cultural values, beliefs, and practices when providing care and support. They should also use a person-centered approach and provide education and support to families and caregivers. Community resources and support are also important for promoting awareness and reducing stigma around the condition. By addressing cultural considerations in dementia care, we can provide more effective and compassionate care for individuals with dementia and their families.

Addressing language barriers and cultural stigma

Dementia is a progressive neurodegenerative disease that can have a significant impact on an individual's ability to communicate and engage in meaningful activities. Providing appropriate care and support for individuals with dementia can be challenging, and it is essential to consider the impact of cultural and linguistic factors on their experience of care. Below we will we will discuss the importance of addressing language barriers and cultural stigma in dementia care and explore strategies for improving cultural competency in dementia care settings.

Language barriers can have a significant impact on the quality of care provided to individuals with dementia. For individuals who do not speak English as their first language, communicating their needs and understanding their care plan can be a daunting task. This can lead to misunderstandings, frustration, and isolation for both the individual and their caregivers. Caregivers must be aware of this challenge and work to provide care that is culturally and linguistically appropriate.

One strategy for addressing language barriers is to provide interpreters or bilingual staff. This can improve communication and facilitate the individual's understanding of their care plan. It is also important to use culturally appropriate communication strategies, such as the use of nonverbal cues or written materials in the individual's native language. Caregivers can also use technology to support communication, such as translation apps or video conferencing with family members who can provide translation.

Cultural stigma surrounding dementia can also be a barrier to providing appropriate care. In some cultures, there may be a belief that dementia is a normal part of aging, or that it is a punishment for past actions. This can lead to individuals and families feeling shame and reluctance to seek help or support. It is important for caregivers to be aware of cultural beliefs and values and to work with families to address any cultural stigma or misconceptions about dementia.

One strategy for addressing cultural stigma is to provide education and awareness programs for individuals and families from diverse cultural backgrounds. These programs can help to increase understanding of dementia, reduce stigma, and provide information on available resources and support. Caregivers can also work with families to develop care plans that respect cultural beliefs and values, while still meeting the individual's needs.

In addition to addressing language barriers and cultural stigma, it is important to consider the impact of cultural diversity on the delivery of care. Cultural competence is the ability to understand, appreciate, and respect the beliefs, values, and practices of individuals from diverse cultures. It is essential for caregivers to be culturally competent to provide appropriate and effective care for individuals with dementia.

One strategy for improving cultural competency in dementia care is to provide cultural competence training for caregivers. This can include education on cultural beliefs and values related to aging and dementia, as well as strategies for providing culturally appropriate care. Caregivers can also engage in ongoing self-reflection and education to improve their understanding of cultural diversity and its impact on care.

Another strategy is to ensure that the care environment is culturally sensitive and welcoming. This can include providing culturally appropriate food, music, and activities, as well as ensuring that the care setting is decorated in a way that is respectful and welcoming to individuals from diverse cultural backgrounds.

In conclusion, addressing language barriers and cultural stigma is essential for providing appropriate and effective care for individuals with dementia. Caregivers must be aware of the impact of cultural and linguistic factors on care and work to provide care that is culturally and linguistically appropriate. Strategies for improving cultural competency in dementia care include providing education and awareness programs, engaging in ongoing self-reflection and education, and ensuring that the care environment is culturally sensitive and welcoming. By working to address these challenges, caregivers can provide high-quality care that respects the beliefs, values, and practices of individuals from diverse cultural backgrounds.

Culturally sensitive care practices

Culturally sensitive care practices are essential in providing high-quality dementia care to individuals from diverse backgrounds. Dementia is a global health issue affecting millions of people worldwide, and it is important to recognize that different cultures may have varying perceptions and beliefs about dementia, which can influence how they respond to and manage the disease. Providing culturally sensitive care can help enhance the patient's quality of life, facilitate communication, and foster mutual respect between healthcare providers, patients, and their families.

One of the key components of culturally sensitive care practices is understanding the cultural norms, values, and beliefs of the patient and their family. This includes recognizing cultural attitudes towards aging, illness, and caregiving, as well as understanding how these beliefs may influence treatment preferences and care decisions. For instance, some cultures place a strong emphasis on family involvement in caregiving, while others may prioritize seeking professional medical help. Healthcare providers must be sensitive to these differences and adapt their approach accordingly.

Effective communication is another essential aspect of culturally sensitive dementia care. Providers must recognize that language barriers can pose significant challenges to effective communication, and they must be prepared to use alternative communication methods, such as interpreters or translation services. Additionally, healthcare providers must be mindful of their own cultural biases and be willing to adapt their communication style to better suit the needs of the patient and their family.

Another critical aspect of culturally sensitive care practices is addressing cultural stigma and misconceptions surrounding dementia. In some cultures, there may be shame or embarrassment associated with cognitive impairment, and patients and families may be reluctant to seek treatment or openly discuss the disease. Healthcare providers must recognize and address these attitudes to ensure that patients receive the care and support they need.

Finally, providing culturally sensitive care also means recognizing and addressing disparities in access to care and resources. In some communities, access to healthcare services and support for dementia patients may be limited, and healthcare providers must be prepared to work with patients and families to find alternative sources of support and care.

In conclusion, providing culturally sensitive care practices is essential in delivering high-quality dementia care to individuals from diverse backgrounds. Understanding cultural norms, values, and beliefs, effective communication, addressing cultural stigma, and addressing disparities in access to care and resources are key components of culturally sensitive care. By implementing these practices, healthcare providers can help enhance the quality of life of dementia patients and their families, foster mutual respect, and improve outcomes.

Chapter Eighteen

Dementia in the LGBTQ+ Community

Dementia is a debilitating disease that affects millions of people worldwide. While the disease can affect anyone regardless of their race, gender, or sexual orientation, studies have shown that individuals who identify as lesbian, gay, bisexual, transgender, or queer (LGBTQ+) may face unique challenges when it comes to dementia care. Below we will we will explore the issues faced by the LGBTQ+ community in relation to dementia and the steps that can be taken to address these challenges.

One of the primary issues faced by the LGBTQ+ community in relation to dementia is a lack of access to culturally sensitive care. The unique experiences and needs of LGBTQ+ individuals are often not addressed in mainstream healthcare settings, which can lead to feelings of isolation, discrimination, and poor quality care. Many LGBTQ+ individuals have experienced discrimination and bias from healthcare providers, which can lead to distrust and reluctance to seek care.

In addition to discrimination from healthcare providers, the LGBTQ+ community may also face discrimination and stigma from family members and caregivers. LGBTQ+ individuals may be estranged from their families, and they may not have access to supportive networks of friends or community members. This lack of support can exacerbate feelings of isolation and can make it difficult for LGBTQ+ individuals to receive the care and support they need.

Furthermore, LGBTQ+ individuals may face unique challenges when it comes to legal and financial planning. Many LGBTQ+ individuals do not have access to legal protections and may face challenges in securing benefits or inheritance rights. This can make it difficult to plan for future care needs and can create additional stress and anxiety for individuals and their caregivers.

To address these challenges, it is important to develop culturally sensitive care practices that are tailored to the needs of the LGBTQ+ community. Healthcare providers must be trained to provide compassionate care that is free from bias and discrimination. Caregivers and family members must also be educated on the unique needs and experiences of LGBTQ+ individuals and should be encouraged to provide supportive care.

One way to address these challenges is through the development of dementia-friendly communities. Dementia-friendly communities aim to create a welcoming and inclusive environment for individuals with dementia and their caregivers. These communities can provide access to supportive services and resources, including legal and financial planning assistance, social programs, and healthcare services.

It is also important to address the issues of stigma and discrimination faced by the LGBTQ+ community. Education and awareness campaigns can help to reduce stigma and promote understanding and acceptance of the LGBTQ+ community. These campaigns can help to create a more supportive and inclusive environment for LGBTQ+ individuals and can encourage greater engagement in healthcare and supportive services.

In conclusion, dementia is a disease that affects individuals from all walks of life, including those who identify as LGBTQ+. The unique challenges faced by the LGBTQ+ community in relation to dementia care must be addressed through the development of culturally sensitive care practices and the creation of dementia-friendly communities. By working to reduce stigma and discrimination and by promoting education and awareness, we can create a more supportive and inclusive environment for all individuals with dementia and their caregivers.

Unique challenges faced by LGBTQ+ individuals with dementia

Dementia is a condition that can affect anyone, regardless of their sexual orientation or gender identity. However, members of the LGBTQ+ community who develop dementia may face unique challenges and barriers when seeking care and support. Below we will explore some of the unique challenges faced by LGBTQ+ individuals with dementia and offer potential solutions to these challenges.

One of the primary challenges faced by LGBTQ+ individuals with dementia is a lack of cultural competency among healthcare providers. Many healthcare providers may not be familiar with the unique needs and experiences of LGBTQ+ individuals, which can lead to inadequate care or even discrimination. For example, LGBTQ+ individuals may have unique health risks and needs that are not always addressed in a healthcare setting, such as increased rates of tobacco use, substance abuse, and mental health issues.

Another challenge faced by LGBTQ+ individuals with dementia is a lack of social support. Due to a history of discrimination and marginalization, many members of the LGBTQ+ community may have limited social networks and may not have close relationships with family members. This can make it challenging for LGBTQ+ individuals with dementia to access the emotional and physical support they need to manage their condition.

Transgender individuals with dementia may face additional challenges related to their gender identity. For example, they may experience discomfort or confusion when being referred to by their birth name or gender. This can be especially distressing for transgender individuals with dementia who may not remember or understand their gender identity. Additionally, transgender individuals with dementia may face challenges related to access to hormones or gender-affirming surgeries.

So how can we address these challenges and ensure that LGBTQ+ individuals with dementia receive the care and support they need? One potential solution is to increase cultural competency among healthcare providers. Healthcare providers can receive training on the unique needs and experiences of LGBTQ+ individuals, including the health risks and barriers to care that they may face. This can help to ensure that healthcare providers are better equipped to provide compassionate and appropriate care to LGBTQ+ individuals with dementia.

Another potential solution is to increase social support for LGBTQ+ individuals with dementia. This can involve connecting individuals with dementia to LGBTQ+-affirming support groups or resources that can provide them with the emotional and physical support they need. Additionally, healthcare providers can work to create safe and welcoming environments for LGBTQ+ individuals with dementia, where they can feel comfortable and supported.

For transgender individuals with dementia, it is important to ensure that their gender identity is respected and affirmed. Healthcare providers can work with transgender individuals with dementia to ensure that they are referred to by their correct name and pronouns, and they can work to ensure that these individuals have access to gender-affirming care when necessary.

In conclusion, dementia can be a challenging and isolating condition for anyone, but LGBTQ+ individuals with dementia may face unique challenges related to cultural competency, social support, and gender identity. By increasing cultural competency among healthcare providers, increasing social support for LGBTQ+ individuals with dementia, and affirming the gender identities of transgender individuals with dementia, we can work to ensure that all individuals with dementia receive the care and support they need.

Affirming and inclusive care practices

Dementia is a complex and challenging disease that affects millions of people worldwide. For members of the LGBTQ+ community, this diagnosis can bring unique challenges and difficulties. Not only do they face the same challenges as the general population, but they also must navigate a healthcare system that may not be inclusive or affirming of their identities.

One of the primary challenges faced by LGBTQ+ individuals with dementia is a lack of social support. Due to stigma and discrimination, many members of this community may have fewer family members or friends to rely on for caregiving and emotional support. This can exacerbate feelings of isolation and loneliness, which are already common in those with dementia.

Another challenge is the lack of culturally competent care. Many healthcare professionals may not have adequate training in providing care to LGBTQ+ individuals, leading to misunderstandings and inappropriate treatment. For example, healthcare professionals may not be familiar with gender-affirming care for transgender individuals or may not understand the importance of using a person's correct pronouns.

The intersection of dementia and HIV/AIDS is another important consideration for the LGBTQ+ community. Many people living with HIV/AIDS are now aging and may be at increased risk for developing dementia. This population may require specialized care and support that takes into account their unique medical history and needs.

To address these challenges, it is essential to create dementia care practices that are affirming and inclusive of LGBTQ+ individuals. This includes training healthcare professionals in culturally competent care, providing social support to LGBTQ+ individuals and their caregivers, and advocating for policies that promote equality and inclusion in healthcare settings.

One important step is to create a welcoming and inclusive environment for LGBTQ+ individuals with dementia. This may include displaying LGBTQ+ symbols and posters in healthcare facilities, using inclusive language in patient interactions, and ensuring that healthcare professionals are trained in providing culturally competent care.

Caregivers and healthcare professionals can also work to build trust and rapport with LGBTQ+ individuals by listening to their needs and concerns and addressing any misunderstandings or miscommunications promptly. It is essential to create a safe and supportive space for individuals to express themselves and their unique needs.

Finally, it is crucial to advocate for policies and programs that promote equality and inclusion in healthcare settings. This may include lobbying for increased funding for culturally competent care and support services, pushing for anti-discrimination laws and policies, and working to ensure that healthcare professionals receive training in LGBTQ+ cultural competence.

In conclusion, dementia is a challenging and complex disease that affects millions of people worldwide. For members of the LGBTQ+ community, this diagnosis can bring unique challenges and difficulties. It is essential to create dementia care practices that are affirming and inclusive of LGBTQ+ individuals. By providing culturally competent care, social support, and advocating for policies that promote equality and inclusion, we can create a more supportive and affirming healthcare system for all individuals affected by dementia.

Resources and support for LGBTQ+ individuals and families

Dementia is a complex and challenging condition that affects millions of people worldwide. For those in the LGBTQ+ community, navigating the experience of dementia can be even more complex due to unique challenges related to identity, stigma, and discrimination. However, there are resources and support available to help LGBTQ+ individuals and their families navigate this difficult journey with dignity and respect.

One of the key challenges faced by LGBTQ+ individuals with dementia is the potential loss of their sense of identity. For many LGBTQ+ individuals, their sense of self is closely tied to their sexual orientation, gender identity, and the communities they belong to. As dementia progresses, individuals may experience memory loss, confusion, and changes in behavior, which can impact their ability to communicate and engage with their communities.

Additionally, LGBTQ+ individuals with dementia may face unique challenges related to stigma and discrimination. Despite increasing acceptance and legal protections for LGBTQ+ individuals, discrimination and prejudice still exist in many parts of the world. For individuals with dementia, discrimination and prejudice can manifest in many forms, including barriers to accessing healthcare, social isolation, and even abuse.

To address these challenges, it is essential for dementia care providers to offer affirming and inclusive care practices. This includes creating a welcoming environment that recognizes and values diverse identities, using appropriate pronouns and terminology, and understanding the unique challenges faced by LGBTQ+ individuals with dementia.

Another important aspect of dementia care for LGBTQ+ individuals is providing access to resources and support. This may include LGBTQ+-specific support groups, counseling services, and legal resources to address discrimination and mistreatment. Families and caregivers of LGBTQ+ individuals with dementia may also benefit from support groups and educational resources to help them navigate the unique challenges of caring for a loved one with dementia.

One organization that offers resources and support for LGBTQ+ individuals with dementia and their families is SAGE. SAGE is a national organization that advocates for LGBTQ+ elders and provides a range of services, including support groups, counseling, and legal resources. The Alzheimer's Association is another organization that offers resources and support for individuals with dementia and their families, including specific resources for LGBTQ+ individuals.

In addition to accessing resources and support, there are also steps that individuals and families can take to promote the well-being of LGBTQ+ individuals with dementia. This includes promoting social connectedness, encouraging engagement with LGBTQ+ communities, and advocating for LGBTQ+-inclusive healthcare services.

In conclusion, dementia can be a challenging and complex experience for anyone, but the unique challenges faced by LGBTQ+ individuals must be acknowledged and addressed. By providing affirming and inclusive care practices, offering resources and support, and promoting social connectedness, individuals and families can navigate the experience of dementia with dignity and respect. It is important that healthcare providers, families, and communities work together to ensure that all individuals with dementia are able to receive the care and support they need to live their lives to the fullest.

Chapter Nineteen

Dementia Research and Advocacy

Dementia is a progressive brain disorder that affects a person's memory, thinking, and behavior. It is estimated that more than 50 million people worldwide have dementia, and this number is expected to triple by 2050. As the population ages, the need for research and advocacy on behalf of those affected by dementia becomes increasingly important. Below we will we will discuss the current state of dementia research and advocacy and the various ways in which individuals and organizations are working to improve the lives of those affected by this condition.

Dementia research has come a long way in recent years, but there is still much to learn about the causes, prevention, and treatment of this condition. One of the biggest challenges in dementia research is the complexity of the brain and the many different types of dementia. Alzheimer's disease is the most common form of dementia, accounting for 60-80% of cases, but there are also many other types, including vascular dementia, Lewy body dementia, and frontotemporal dementia.

Despite these challenges, there has been significant progress in dementia research in recent years. Researchers have made great strides in identifying genetic and environmental factors that may contribute to the development of dementia. They have also made progress in developing new drugs and treatments to slow or even reverse the progression of dementia. For example, the drug aducanumab was recently approved by the FDA for the treatment of Alzheimer's disease. While this is a significant step forward, more research is needed to fully understand the drug's efficacy and potential side effects.

In addition to research, advocacy is also an important component of the fight against dementia. Advocacy can take many different forms, from raising awareness to lobbying for policy changes to providing support to those affected by dementia. One of the most important advocacy efforts in the fight against dementia is the push for increased funding for research. Without adequate funding, progress in dementia research will be slow, and new treatments and cures will be more difficult to develop.

Another important aspect of dementia advocacy is raising awareness about the condition and its impact on individuals, families, and communities. This includes educating the public about the signs and symptoms of dementia, as well as the resources available for those affected by the condition. It also involves challenging the stigma surrounding dementia and promoting a more inclusive and supportive society for those living with the condition.

Organizations such as the Alzheimer's Association and the Dementia Alliance International play a critical role in both dementia research and advocacy. These organizations work to raise awareness, provide support and resources for those affected by dementia, and advocate for policy changes and increased funding for research.

One of the most exciting developments in dementia research is the focus on prevention and early intervention. Researchers have identified several risk factors for dementia, including high blood pressure, high cholesterol, diabetes, and obesity. By addressing these risk factors early on, it may be possible to reduce the risk of developing dementia later in life. Additionally, early intervention with cognitive training and lifestyle changes may also help slow the progression of dementia in those already affected by the condition.

In conclusion, dementia research and advocacy are critical components of the fight against this devastating condition. While there has been significant progress in recent years, there is still much work to be done. Continued research and advocacy efforts are needed to better understand the causes, prevention, and treatment of dementia, and to improve the lives of those affected by the condition. By working together, we can create a brighter future for all those affected by dementia.

Current research and clinical trials

Dementia is a complex and debilitating disease that affects millions of people worldwide. While there is currently no cure for dementia, ongoing research and clinical trials offer hope for better treatments and ultimately a cure. Below we will we will explore some of the current research and clinical trials related to dementia.

One area of research focuses on identifying early signs of dementia. Early detection is essential for the development of effective treatments that can slow or stop the progression of the disease. Researchers are exploring a range of approaches to identify early signs of dementia, including brain imaging, blood tests, and cognitive testing. Some studies are also investigating the use of artificial intelligence to identify subtle changes in brain function that may indicate the onset of dementia.

Another area of research is focused on developing new treatments for dementia. There are currently no drugs that can cure or stop the progression of dementia, and existing treatments can only alleviate symptoms. Researchers are exploring a range of approaches, including drugs that target the buildup of abnormal proteins in the brain, anti-inflammatory drugs, and stem cell therapy. Many of these approaches are still in the early stages of development, but there is hope that they may one day lead to effective treatments.

Clinical trials are a crucial part of the research process, providing an opportunity to test new treatments in humans. There are currently numerous clinical trials underway, testing a range of treatments for dementia. One promising trial is investigating the use of a drug called aducanumab to target the buildup of amyloid plaques in the brain, which are associated with Alzheimer's disease. Results from early studies have shown promising results, with the drug appearing to slow the progression of the disease in some patients.

Another clinical trial is exploring the use of deep brain stimulation to treat the symptoms of Alzheimer's disease. Deep brain stimulation involves the implantation of electrodes in the brain, which deliver electrical impulses to targeted areas. While the approach has been used successfully to treat conditions such as Parkinson's disease, its use in dementia is still in the early stages of investigation.

Research is also exploring the role of lifestyle factors in the development and progression of dementia. Studies have shown that factors such as exercise, diet, and social interaction can play a significant role in reducing the risk of developing dementia. Researchers are also exploring the use of non-pharmacological interventions, such as cognitive training and music therapy, to alleviate symptoms of dementia and improve quality of life for patients.

Advocacy is another critical area of focus in dementia research. Advocacy groups play an essential role in raising awareness of the disease, advocating for funding for research and support services, and providing resources and support to patients and their families. The Alzheimer's Association is one such group, offering a range of services and resources, including support groups, educational materials, and advocacy initiatives.

In conclusion, while there is currently no cure for dementia, ongoing research and clinical trials offer hope for better treatments and ultimately a cure. Researchers are exploring a range of approaches, from early detection to lifestyle interventions and new drugs. Clinical trials are crucial in the development of new treatments, and advocacy groups play a vital role in raising awareness and advocating for funding and support services. While much work remains to be done, the progress being made in dementia research is cause for optimism.

Advocacy organizations and initiatives

Advocacy organizations and initiatives play a crucial role in raising awareness and advocating for individuals with dementia and their families. These organizations work towards improving the lives of those living with dementia by providing education, resources, and support, and advocating for policy changes at the local, national, and global levels.

One of the largest advocacy organizations in the United States is the Alzheimer's Association, which was founded in 1980. The Alzheimer's Association is dedicated to providing education, support, and advocacy to individuals living with Alzheimer's disease and other forms of dementia, as well as their families and caregivers. The organization offers a range of services, including a 24/7 helpline, support groups, care consultations, and educational programs for healthcare professionals and the general public. Additionally, the Alzheimer's Association is actively involved in advocacy efforts to increase funding for research and to improve policies related to dementia care.

Another major advocacy organization is the Dementia Action Alliance, which is focused on promoting person-centered care and empowering individuals with dementia to have a voice in their care. The Dementia Action Alliance provides education and training to healthcare professionals and caregivers on person-centered care, and also hosts conferences and events to raise awareness about dementia and the need for person-centered care. The organization also provides support to individuals with dementia and their families, and advocates for policy changes that prioritize person-centered care.

In addition to these national organizations, there are also a number of smaller advocacy groups that focus on specific populations or issues related to dementia. For example, the Lewy Body Dementia Association is dedicated to raising awareness about Lewy body dementia and providing education and support to individuals with the condition and their families. The National Hispanic Council on Aging works to address the unique needs and challenges faced by Hispanic/Latino individuals with dementia and their families, while the LGBT Elder Initiative focuses on promoting culturally sensitive care and support for LGBT individuals with dementia.

Advocacy organizations also play a critical role in advocating for policy changes related to dementia care. For example, the Alzheimer's Impact Movement is the advocacy arm of the Alzheimer's Association, and works to advance policies at the federal level that will improve care and support for individuals with dementia and their families. This includes advocating for increased funding for research, improving access to care and support services, and expanding access to clinical trials for individuals with dementia.

The Global Alzheimer's and Dementia Action Alliance is another international organization that works towards improving dementia care and support around the world. The organization brings together a range of stakeholders, including individuals with dementia, caregivers, healthcare professionals, and policy makers, to collaborate and advocate for policy changes that prioritize dementia care and support.

In addition to these advocacy organizations, there are also a number of initiatives focused on advancing dementia research and improving care and support for individuals with dementia. The National Plan to Address Alzheimer's Disease is a government initiative launched in 2012 to accelerate progress in Alzheimer's research and care. The plan includes a range of goals and strategies aimed at improving the understanding and treatment of Alzheimer's disease, and increasing access to care and support services for individuals with the condition and their families.

The Dementia Discovery Fund is another initiative focused on advancing dementia research. The fund is a venture capital fund that invests in innovative research projects aimed at developing new treatments and therapies for dementia. The fund has invested in a range of research areas, including drug discovery, genetics, and digital health technologies.

Overall, advocacy organizations and initiatives play a crucial role in advancing dementia research, improving care and support for individuals with dementia and their families, and advocating for policy changes at the local, national, and global levels. Through education, resources, support, and advocacy, these organizations and initiatives are working towards a future where individuals with dementia can receive the care and support they need to live well with the condition.

The role of public policy in dementia care

Dementia is a significant health issue that affects millions of people worldwide. As the global population ages, dementia cases are projected to increase dramatically. As such, it is essential that public policy makers prioritize dementia care and establish policies that promote better care for those living with dementia.

One of the key roles of public policy in dementia care is to promote awareness of the condition and its impact on individuals and society as a whole. This includes raising awareness of the warning signs of dementia, as well as the importance of early diagnosis and treatment. Public policy can help support campaigns to increase public understanding of dementia, reduce stigma associated with the condition, and encourage people to seek medical care.

In addition to raising awareness, public policy plays a critical role in providing support for people with dementia and their families. This includes ensuring access to high-quality healthcare, home care services, and community-based programs that provide social and emotional support. Public policy can help ensure that these services are affordable and accessible to all who need them, regardless of their socioeconomic status or geographic location.

Public policy also plays a vital role in supporting dementia research. Through funding and regulation, policy makers can promote research aimed at understanding the causes of dementia, developing new treatments, and improving care for those living with the condition. This includes research into non-pharmacological interventions, such as music therapy and art therapy, which have been shown to have a positive impact on the quality of life of people with dementia.

Another critical area where public policy can have a positive impact on dementia care is in promoting dementia-friendly communities. A dementia-friendly community is one that is supportive and welcoming to people with dementia and their families. This includes ensuring that public spaces are accessible and safe, providing training for businesses and service providers to better understand the needs of people with dementia, and promoting social inclusion.

Finally, public policy plays a critical role in addressing the financial burden of dementia care. As the cost of care for people with dementia continues to rise, many families are left struggling to cover the costs of care. Public policy can help address this by promoting the development of new funding mechanisms, such as tax credits and subsidies, that can help offset the cost of care.

In conclusion, public policy plays a vital role in dementia care. Through funding, regulation, and awareness campaigns, public policy can help promote better care for people with dementia, support their families, and promote dementia-friendly communities. With the number of dementia cases projected to rise in the coming years, it is essential that policy makers prioritize dementia care and work to establish policies that promote better care and support for those living with the condition.

Chapter Twenty

Ethics and Dementia

Dementia is a complex and progressive condition that affects an individual's ability to think, remember, and communicate. As the disease progresses, individuals with dementia may become increasingly dependent on others for support and care. As a result, ethical considerations are an important aspect of dementia care that should be taken into account. Below we will explore the ethical issues surrounding dementia and discuss the different approaches to ethical decision-making in dementia care.

One of the most significant ethical considerations in dementia care is autonomy. Autonomy refers to an individual's right to make decisions about their own life and health care. As the disease progresses, individuals with dementia may lose their ability to make informed decisions about their care. This loss of autonomy can present significant ethical challenges for caregivers, who must balance the individual's right to make decisions with the need to ensure their safety and well-being.

Another ethical consideration in dementia care is the need to respect the individual's dignity and quality of life. Individuals with dementia may experience feelings of confusion, frustration, and isolation. Caregivers must ensure that these individuals are treated with respect and that their quality of life is maximized to the extent possible. This may involve providing social stimulation, promoting physical activity, and ensuring that the individual's basic needs are met.

The issue of informed consent is also a significant ethical consideration in dementia care. Informed consent refers to an individual's right to be fully informed about their care and to make decisions based on this information. As the disease progresses, individuals with dementia may lose their ability to understand and retain complex medical information. This can make it difficult for caregivers to obtain informed consent for medical treatments or procedures.

The use of restraints is another ethical consideration in dementia care. Restraints are physical devices or medications used to restrict an individual's movement or behavior. While restraints can be effective in preventing injury or harm, they can also limit an individual's autonomy and dignity. In addition, the use of restraints can increase the risk of injury or death, particularly in individuals with dementia who may become agitated or confused.

One approach to ethical decision-making in dementia care is the use of advance directives. Advance directives are legal documents that allow individuals to express their preferences for medical treatment in the event that they become incapacitated. By completing an advance directive, individuals with dementia can ensure that their wishes regarding their care are respected, even if they are no longer able to make decisions for themselves.

Another approach to ethical decision-making in dementia care is the use of a care team. A care team is a group of professionals who work together to develop a comprehensive care plan for individuals with dementia. The care team may include physicians, nurses, social workers, and other healthcare professionals. By working together, the care team can ensure that the individual's needs and preferences are taken into account, and that ethical considerations are addressed in a timely and appropriate manner.

In conclusion, dementia presents significant ethical considerations for caregivers and healthcare professionals. Autonomy, dignity, informed consent, the use of restraints, and advance directives are all important issues to consider when caring for individuals with dementia. By using approaches such as advance directives and care teams, caregivers can ensure that the individual's needs and preferences are taken into account, and that ethical considerations are addressed in a timely and appropriate manner. Ultimately, ethical decision-making in dementia care requires a balance between respecting the individual's autonomy and ensuring their safety and well-being.

Ethical considerations in dementia care

Dementia is a condition that affects millions of people worldwide, and it poses many ethical challenges for caregivers and healthcare professionals. As the condition progresses, individuals with dementia may lose their ability to make decisions, communicate effectively, and participate in their own care. This loss of autonomy raises important ethical questions about the balance between respecting a person's autonomy and ensuring their safety and well-being.

One of the most significant ethical issues in dementia care is the decision-making process. As dementia progresses, individuals may lose their ability to make decisions about their care, finances, and other important aspects of their life. This can be particularly challenging for caregivers and family members who must make decisions on behalf of their loved one. There are often questions about who should make these decisions and how much authority they should have.

The principle of autonomy is one of the guiding ethical principles in healthcare, which means that individuals have the right to make their own decisions. However, this principle can conflict with the principle of beneficence, which requires healthcare providers to act in the best interests of their patients. In the case of dementia care, the ethical challenge is to balance the patient's autonomy with the need to ensure their safety and well-being.

Another ethical issue in dementia care is the use of restraints and medications. Some individuals with dementia may become agitated, aggressive, or otherwise difficult to manage, leading some caregivers and healthcare providers to consider the use of restraints or medications to control their behavior. However, these interventions raise ethical questions about the use of force and the potential side effects of medications.

The use of restraints is a controversial issue in dementia care, and it is generally discouraged due to the risk of injury and the potential loss of autonomy for the patient. Similarly, medications such as antipsychotics and sedatives can have significant side effects, including cognitive impairment, falls, and increased mortality risk. The ethical challenge for healthcare providers is to balance the need to manage difficult behaviors with the potential harm caused by these interventions.

Finally, there are ethical considerations related to end-of-life care in individuals with dementia. As the condition progresses, individuals may reach a point where they can no longer communicate their wishes about end-of-life care. In these cases, family members and healthcare providers must make decisions about the appropriate level of care, including palliative care and hospice care.

The ethical challenge in end-of-life care is to ensure that the patient's wishes and values are respected, even if they are unable to communicate them. Healthcare providers must also consider the impact of these decisions on the patient's family members and caregivers.

To address these ethical challenges in dementia care, healthcare providers and caregivers must consider the principles of autonomy, beneficence, non-maleficence, and justice. Autonomy means respecting the patient's right to make their own decisions, while beneficence requires healthcare providers to act in the patient's best interests. Non-maleficence means avoiding harm to the patient, and justice means treating all patients fairly and without discrimination.

In addition to these principles, healthcare providers and caregivers should also be aware of the ethical guidelines and recommendations provided by professional organizations such as the Alzheimer's Association and the National Institute on Aging. These organizations provide guidance on a wide range of ethical issues related to dementia care, including decision-making, end-of-life care, and the use of medications and restraints.

In conclusion, dementia presents many ethical challenges for healthcare providers and caregivers, including decision-making, the use of restraints and medications, and end-of-life care. To address these challenges, it is essential to balance the principles of autonomy, beneficence, non-maleficence, and justice while following the ethical guidelines and recommendations provided by professional organizations.

Informed consent and decision-making

Informed consent and decision-making are important ethical considerations in dementia care. Dementia is a progressive disorder that affects a person's cognitive abilities, leading to memory loss, impaired judgment, and difficulty with communication. This can make decision-making and informed consent challenging for individuals with dementia, as well as their caregivers and healthcare providers.

Informed consent is the process of obtaining permission from a patient or their surrogate decision-maker before proceeding with a medical intervention or treatment. Informed consent requires that the patient has the capacity to make decisions and has been provided with adequate information about the risks and benefits of the proposed intervention or treatment. However, in dementia care, capacity may be impaired, making it difficult for patients to understand and make decisions about their care.

In these situations, surrogate decision-makers, such as family members or legally appointed guardians, may make decisions on behalf of the patient. Surrogates must act in the patient's best interests, taking into account their wishes, values, and beliefs, as well as any prior expressed preferences or advance directives. In addition, healthcare providers should provide information in a way that is understandable and meaningful to the patient and their surrogate decision-maker.

It is important to note that ethical considerations in dementia care are not limited to medical decision-making. Dementia can impact a person's ability to make decisions about their finances, living arrangements, and social relationships. Caregivers and healthcare providers must work together to ensure that the person with dementia is supported in all areas of their life and that their autonomy and dignity are respected.

One approach to promoting informed consent and decision-making in dementia care is through shared decision-making. Shared decision-making involves collaboration between the patient, their caregiver, and their healthcare provider to make decisions that align with the patient's goals, preferences, and values. This approach emphasizes the importance of communication and trust between all parties involved and aims to ensure that the patient's voice is heard and respected.

Another important consideration in dementia care is the use of advance directives, such as a living will or durable power of attorney for healthcare. These documents allow individuals to express their preferences for medical treatment and appoint a surrogate decision-maker in the event that they are unable to make decisions for themselves. Advance directives can provide important guidance for healthcare providers and caregivers in making decisions that align with the patient's wishes.

However, it is important to note that advance directives may not always be applicable in the context of dementia care. As dementia progresses, a person's wishes and values may change, and their ability to communicate these changes may be impaired. In these situations, healthcare providers and surrogate decision-makers must use their best judgment to make decisions that align with the person's best interests.

In conclusion, informed consent and decision-making are important ethical considerations in dementia care. These considerations are complex, and they require collaboration between the patient, their caregivers, and their healthcare providers. The use of shared decision-making, advance directives, and careful communication can promote autonomy and dignity for individuals with dementia, while also ensuring that they receive appropriate and compassionate care.

The debate over assisted dying and dementia

The debate over assisted dying and dementia is a complex and controversial issue that raises questions about ethics, autonomy, and the value of life. Dementia is a progressive and irreversible brain disorder that affects millions of people worldwide. As the disease advances, individuals with dementia may lose their capacity to make decisions about their own care and may experience significant suffering. For some, the prospect of living with advanced dementia is unbearable, and they may wish to end their lives on their own terms.

Assisted dying, also known as euthanasia or physician-assisted suicide, is the intentional ending of a person's life with the assistance of a healthcare professional. This practice is legal in a few countries and states, but remains controversial and illegal in many others. In the context of dementia, assisted dying is particularly controversial because of the challenges in assessing an individual's capacity to make a decision about ending their own life, as well as concerns about protecting vulnerable individuals from abuse and coercion.

Those who support assisted dying for individuals with dementia argue that it is a compassionate response to the suffering that individuals with advanced dementia may experience. They believe that individuals with dementia should have the right to choose to end their lives if they are no longer able to enjoy their lives and are experiencing significant physical or emotional pain. Supporters also argue that assisted dying may help to reduce the burden on caregivers and healthcare systems by allowing individuals to die on their own terms.

Opponents of assisted dying for individuals with dementia argue that it is ethically and morally wrong to intentionally end a person's life, regardless of the circumstances. They believe that every life is valuable and that assisted dying sends the message that some lives are not worth living. Opponents also argue that there is a risk of abuse and coercion in the context of dementia, particularly given the vulnerability of individuals with the disease and the potential for family members or caregivers to pressure them into making a decision to end their lives.

In addition to the ethical and moral considerations, there are also practical challenges in implementing assisted dying for individuals with dementia.

One of the main challenges is assessing an individual's capacity to make a decision about ending their own life. Dementia is a progressive disease that affects cognitive function, and individuals with advanced dementia may not be able to understand the consequences of their decision or communicate their wishes effectively. This raises concerns about the possibility of individuals with dementia being coerced or manipulated into making a decision that they do not fully understand.

Another challenge is ensuring that the decision to end a person's life is truly voluntary and not influenced by external factors such as financial pressure or a lack of access to quality care. Given the stigma and lack of support for individuals with dementia and their families, there is a risk that assisted dying could become a default option rather than a truly voluntary choice.

Finally, there are concerns about the impact of assisted dying on the broader society and the message that it sends about the value of life. Critics argue that legalizing assisted dying for individuals with dementia could contribute to a culture that devalues the lives of older adults and people with disabilities, and that it could lead to a slippery slope in which assisted dying is extended to other groups of people.

In conclusion, the debate over assisted dying and dementia is a complex and multifaceted issue that raises important questions about ethics, autonomy, and the value of life. While supporters of assisted dying argue that it is a compassionate response to the suffering of individuals with dementia, opponents argue that it is ethically and morally wrong to intentionally end a person's life. In addition to these ethical and moral considerations, there are also practical challenges in implementing assisted dying for individuals with dementia, particularly in assessing an individual's capacity to make a decision and ensuring that the decision is truly voluntary.

Chapter Twenty-One

Personal Stories and Experiences

Dementia is a condition that affects millions of people worldwide, and its impact is not limited to the individuals diagnosed with it. Family members, friends, and caregivers are also greatly affected by the disease. Personal stories and experiences of those affected by dementia can help others understand the challenges and difficulties associated with the disease, and provide a platform for advocacy and awareness.

One of the most significant challenges of dementia is the progressive loss of memory and cognitive function. This can lead to a sense of disorientation and confusion, making it difficult for individuals to carry out day-to-day tasks. In addition, dementia can also lead to changes in behavior, mood swings, and difficulty with communication. For caregivers, this can be particularly challenging, as they often have to adjust their own schedules and routines to provide care and support for their loved ones.

Personal stories and experiences of those affected by dementia can provide insight into the emotional toll of the disease. For example, individuals with dementia may feel frustrated, angry, or scared as they struggle to maintain their independence and sense of self. Caregivers may also experience a range of emotions, including guilt, stress, and anxiety as they try to balance their own needs with the needs of their loved ones.

One of the most significant benefits of sharing personal stories and experiences is that it can help reduce the stigma associated with dementia.

Many people may feel ashamed or embarrassed about their diagnosis or may not want to talk about it. However, by sharing their experiences, individuals with dementia and their caregivers can help raise awareness and educate others about the disease. This can help reduce the isolation and loneliness that can often accompany the disease, and encourage others to seek support and resources.

In addition, personal stories and experiences can also serve as a source of hope and inspiration. Many individuals with dementia and their caregivers have found ways to cope with the challenges of the disease and maintain a sense of joy and purpose in their lives. These stories can serve as a reminder that there is life beyond dementia, and that individuals with the disease can still lead fulfilling lives.

There are many ways in which individuals and organizations can share personal stories and experiences related to dementia. One way is through support groups and online forums, where individuals can connect with others who are going through similar experiences. Many organizations also offer storytelling events or workshops, where individuals can share their stories with a wider audience.

In recent years, there has been a growing movement to incorporate personal stories and experiences into dementia care and research. For example, some healthcare professionals are using storytelling as a therapeutic tool to help individuals with dementia express themselves and connect with others. In addition, researchers are also studying the impact of personal stories and experiences on caregiver well-being and the effectiveness of interventions designed to support individuals with dementia and their families.

In conclusion, personal stories and experiences play an important role in dementia advocacy, awareness, and research. By sharing their experiences, individuals with dementia and their caregivers can help reduce stigma, raise awareness, and inspire others. As the world continues to grapple with the challenges of dementia, it is important to recognize the power of personal stories and experiences to inform and inspire change.

First-hand accounts of living with dementia

Dementia is a progressive neurological disorder that affects memory, thinking, and behavior. It can be a frightening and isolating experience for those living with the disease and their families. However, first-hand accounts from people with dementia can provide valuable insights and help others understand the experience of living with the disease.

One of the most common experiences shared by people with dementia is the loss of memory. Many describe feeling frustrated and confused when they cannot remember important information such as their own name or where they live. This loss of memory can also affect the ability to recognize loved ones and can cause feelings of loneliness and isolation.

Communication can also be challenging for people with dementia. As the disease progresses, it can become difficult to find the right words or to follow a conversation. This can be frustrating for both the person with dementia and their loved ones, who may feel like they are not being heard or understood.

The loss of independence is another common experience shared by those with dementia. As the disease progresses, it can become more difficult to perform everyday tasks such as dressing, grooming, and cooking. This loss of independence can be challenging and can lead to feelings of helplessness and frustration.

Despite the challenges of living with dementia, many people with the disease remain positive and focused on living their lives to the fullest. They may find new hobbies or ways to express themselves creatively, such as through painting, writing, or music. Others may choose to participate in support groups or advocate for better care and support for people with dementia.

Family members and caregivers of those with dementia can also learn from first-hand accounts. They can gain a better understanding of the challenges faced by their loved one and may be able to offer more compassionate care and support.

It is important to remember that each person's experience with dementia is unique. Some may experience more severe symptoms than others, and the progression of the disease can vary widely. However, first-hand accounts can help to break down the stigma surrounding dementia and increase awareness of the challenges faced by those with the disease.

There are many resources available for people with dementia and their families, including support groups, counseling services, and educational programs. These resources can provide valuable information and help people connect with others who are going through similar experiences.

In conclusion, first-hand accounts of living with dementia can provide valuable insights into the experience of the disease. They can help to break down the stigma surrounding dementia and increase awareness of the challenges faced by those with the disease. By listening to and learning from the experiences of people with dementia, we can work towards better care and support for those living with the disease and their families.

Caregiver perspectives and insights

Caring for someone with dementia can be a challenging and emotionally demanding experience for family members and other caregivers. Providing support, patience, and understanding can make a significant difference in the quality of life for both the person with dementia and their caregiver. Caregivers of people with dementia can offer unique insights into the needs of the person they care for and the challenges they face. Below we will we will explore the perspectives and insights of caregivers and the importance of their role in dementia care.

Caregivers are often the primary source of support for people with dementia. They provide personal care, emotional support, and practical assistance with daily activities such as bathing, dressing, and eating. They also help manage the person's medical care, medications, and appointments. Caregivers may also be responsible for managing finances, legal affairs, and other aspects of daily living. The demands of caregiving can be overwhelming, and caregivers may experience stress, burnout, and other health problems as a result.

One of the most significant challenges faced by caregivers of people with dementia is managing the person's behaviors and mood changes. Dementia can cause changes in behavior, such as aggression, wandering, and agitation, which can be difficult to manage. Caregivers must learn to respond calmly and positively to these behaviors while also keeping the person safe. They must also adapt to the person's changing mood, which may include depression, anxiety, or apathy. Caregivers must be patient, flexible, and willing to adapt to the person's needs.

Another challenge for caregivers is the isolation and loneliness that can come with caring for someone with dementia. Caregivers may feel overwhelmed by the demands of caregiving, which can lead to social isolation and a sense of loneliness. They may also feel stigmatized or misunderstood by others who do not understand the challenges of caring for someone with dementia. Caregivers must find ways to stay connected with others and maintain a sense of purpose and meaning in their lives.

Despite the challenges, many caregivers find that caring for someone with dementia is a rewarding experience. They may feel a sense of purpose and fulfillment in providing care and support to someone they love. Caregivers also offer unique insights into the needs and experiences of people with dementia. They can help identify the person's preferences, routines, and interests, which can inform their care plan. Caregivers can also help healthcare providers understand the person's behavior and mood changes, which can guide their treatment and support.

Caregivers can also play an essential role in advocating for the needs and rights of people with dementia. They can help raise awareness about the challenges faced by people with dementia and their caregivers and advocate for better access to support services and resources. Caregivers can also share their experiences and insights to help improve dementia care and research.

In conclusion, caregivers are an essential part of dementia care. They provide invaluable support, insight, and advocacy for people with dementia and their families. Caregiving can be a challenging and emotionally demanding experience, but it can also be a rewarding one. Caregivers must find ways to manage the challenges of caregiving while also maintaining their own health and well-being. Caregivers offer a unique perspective that can help inform and improve dementia care and research. By supporting caregivers, we can improve the quality of life for people with dementia and their families.

Inspiring stories of resilience and hope

Dementia can be a devastating diagnosis, not just for the individual who receives it, but for their loved ones as well. It can be a difficult journey filled with challenges, but amidst the struggles, there are also stories of resilience and hope.

One such story is that of Norm Macdonald, the beloved comedian and former Saturday Night Live cast member. In 2018, Macdonald revealed that he had been diagnosed with dementia, specifically a form of the disease called Lewy body dementia. Despite the diagnosis, Macdonald continued to perform stand-up comedy, even incorporating his experience with dementia into his act. He used humor as a way to cope with his illness, and his resilience in the face of such a difficult diagnosis was truly inspiring.

Another inspiring story is that of Pauline Boss, a pioneer in the field of grief and loss. Boss coined the term "ambiguous loss" to describe the unique grief experienced by those caring for loved ones with dementia. This type of loss is different from other types of loss because it involves ongoing uncertainty, as the person with dementia may be physically present but mentally absent. Boss's work has helped many caregivers to better understand their experiences and find ways to cope with the complex emotions that come with caring for a loved one with dementia.

In addition to individual stories, there are also inspiring initiatives and programs that aim to improve the lives of those living with dementia. One such initiative is the Dementia Friendly America program, which seeks to create communities that are more inclusive and supportive of people with dementia. Through this program, communities work to increase awareness and understanding of dementia, as well as to improve accessibility and reduce stigma. By creating more dementia-friendly communities, people with dementia and their caregivers can feel more supported and less isolated.

Another inspiring program is the Alzheimer's Poetry Project, which uses poetry and storytelling to connect with people with dementia and help them express themselves. Through interactive poetry sessions, people with dementia are able to share their memories, feelings, and experiences in a meaningful way. This program has been shown to improve mood and social engagement in people with dementia, and it serves as a reminder that creative expression can be a powerful tool for connecting with others.

Finally, the story of Kate Swaffer, an Australian woman living with dementia, is one of resilience, advocacy, and hope. After being diagnosed with dementia at the age of 49, Swaffer became a vocal advocate for people with dementia, using her own experience to raise awareness and fight for change. She founded the Dementia Alliance International, an organization run by people with dementia for people with dementia, and has become a leading voice in the movement for dementia rights. Swaffer's resilience in the face of such a devastating diagnosis is truly remarkable, and her advocacy work serves as an inspiration to others.

In conclusion, while dementia can be a challenging and difficult journey, there are also stories of resilience and hope that offer inspiration and encouragement. From individuals who use humor and creativity to cope with their illness, to programs and initiatives that aim to create more supportive and inclusive communities, there are many examples of people making a positive impact in the world of dementia care. By sharing these stories and experiences, we can raise awareness of dementia and help others to feel less alone in their journey.

Chapter Twenty-Two

Prevention and Brain Health

Dementia is a progressive neurological disorder that affects cognitive function, memory, and behavior. While there is no known cure for dementia, research has shown that certain lifestyle changes and interventions can help reduce the risk of developing the condition. Additionally, maintaining overall brain health is important in preventing cognitive decline and maintaining cognitive function as we age. Below we will we will explore various prevention strategies and brain health practices that can help reduce the risk of developing dementia.

One of the most important prevention strategies is maintaining a healthy lifestyle. Research has shown that factors such as high blood pressure, high cholesterol, and obesity can increase the risk of developing dementia. Therefore, managing these conditions through diet, exercise, and medication can help reduce the risk of developing the condition. Regular exercise has also been shown to improve cognitive function and memory retention, as well as reduce the risk of developing dementia. Additionally, maintaining a healthy and balanced diet that is rich in fruits, vegetables, and whole grains can help reduce the risk of developing cognitive decline.

Another important prevention strategy is engaging in mentally stimulating activities. Studies have shown that participating in activities that challenge the brain, such as reading, doing puzzles, or playing games, can help improve cognitive function and reduce the risk of developing dementia. Additionally, staying socially engaged and maintaining meaningful relationships with family and friends can also help reduce the risk of developing the condition.

In addition to prevention strategies, there are various brain health practices that can help maintain cognitive function and reduce the risk of developing dementia. One such practice is getting enough sleep. Research has shown that chronic sleep deprivation can lead to cognitive decline, while getting enough restful sleep can help improve cognitive function and reduce the risk of developing dementia.

Another important brain health practice is managing stress. Chronic stress has been linked to cognitive decline, while reducing stress through practices such as meditation or mindfulness can help maintain cognitive function and reduce the risk of developing dementia. Additionally, engaging in hobbies or activities that promote relaxation and calmness, such as yoga or gardening, can also help reduce stress and promote overall brain health.

Finally, it is important to stay mentally active throughout life. This can include learning new skills, taking classes, or engaging in other intellectually stimulating activities. It is important to continue challenging the brain and promoting cognitive function throughout life in order to maintain brain health and reduce the risk of developing dementia.

In conclusion, while there is no known cure for dementia, there are various prevention strategies and brain health practices that can help reduce the risk of developing the condition. These strategies include maintaining a healthy lifestyle, engaging in mentally stimulating activities, getting enough restful sleep, managing stress, and staying mentally active throughout life. By implementing these practices, we can help maintain cognitive function and promote overall brain health, reducing the risk of developing dementia and other cognitive disorders.

Lifestyle factors for reducing dementia risk

Dementia is a debilitating disease that affects millions of people worldwide, and the number of individuals living with dementia is expected to increase in the coming decades. While there is no cure for dementia, there are ways to reduce the risk of developing the disease, and lifestyle factors play a crucial role in dementia prevention. Below we will we will explore the lifestyle factors that can help reduce the risk of developing dementia.

One of the most important lifestyle factors for reducing dementia risk is physical activity. Regular exercise has been shown to reduce the risk of developing dementia by up to 30%. Exercise helps to improve cardiovascular health, which in turn improves brain health. It also helps to increase blood flow to the brain, which can improve cognitive function. Regular exercise can also help to reduce stress and improve mood, which can have a positive impact on brain health.

Another lifestyle factor that can help reduce the risk of developing dementia is a healthy diet. A diet that is rich in fruits, vegetables, whole grains, and lean protein can help to reduce the risk of developing dementia. Some studies suggest that a Mediterranean diet, which includes olive oil, fish, and nuts, may be particularly beneficial for brain health. A healthy diet can also help to reduce the risk of developing other health conditions, such as obesity and diabetes, which are known risk factors for dementia.

In addition to physical activity and a healthy diet, staying socially engaged is another important lifestyle factor for reducing dementia risk. Social interaction has been shown to help maintain cognitive function and reduce the risk of developing dementia. Activities such as volunteering, participating in community events, and staying connected with friends and family can all help to keep the brain healthy and reduce the risk of developing dementia.

Getting enough sleep is also important for reducing dementia risk. Studies have shown that sleep deprivation can have a negative impact on brain function and increase the risk of developing dementia. It is important to get enough sleep each night, and to establish a regular sleep routine to help improve sleep quality.

Finally, it is important to manage chronic health conditions to reduce the risk of developing dementia. Conditions such as high blood pressure, diabetes, and high cholesterol can all increase the risk of developing dementia. By managing these conditions and keeping them under control, individuals can help to reduce their risk of developing dementia.

In conclusion, there are several lifestyle factors that can help reduce the risk of developing dementia. Physical activity, a healthy diet, social engagement, getting enough sleep, and managing chronic health conditions can all have a positive impact on brain health and reduce the risk of developing dementia. While there is no sure way to prevent dementia, incorporating these lifestyle factors into daily life can help to maintain cognitive function and reduce the risk of developing this debilitating disease.

Cognitive stimulation and brain training

As people age, they may become more concerned about cognitive decline and the potential onset of dementia. While there is currently no known cure for dementia, there are steps that can be taken to help reduce the risk of developing it. One such step is cognitive stimulation and brain training.

Cognitive stimulation refers to activities that engage the brain and promote mental activity. These activities can include anything from playing games and puzzles to reading and socializing. Brain training, on the other hand, involves specific exercises designed to improve cognitive function and strengthen neural connections in the brain.

Research has shown that both cognitive stimulation and brain training can have positive effects on cognitive function and may help reduce the risk of developing dementia. In one study, participants who engaged in cognitive stimulation activities had a lower risk of developing dementia over a four-year period than those who did not. In another study, participants who engaged in brain training exercises showed improvements in memory and cognitive function.

So, what are some effective ways to engage in cognitive stimulation and brain training? Here are a few ideas:

1. Play games and puzzles: Games and puzzles, such as crossword puzzles, Sudoku, and card games, can be fun and engaging ways to stimulate the brain. These activities can help improve memory, problem-solving skills, and attention.

2. Read and learn: Reading and learning new things can help keep the brain active and engaged. Consider joining a book club or taking a class in a subject you are interested in.

3. Stay socially active: Socializing and engaging with others can help keep the brain active and reduce the risk of isolation and depression, which can contribute to cognitive decline. Consider joining a social club or volunteering in your community.

4. Exercise: Physical exercise has been shown to have positive effects on brain health and cognitive function. Aim for at least 30 minutes of exercise per day, such as brisk walking, swimming, or yoga.

5. Try brain training exercises: There are many brain training exercises available, both online and through apps. These exercises are designed to improve cognitive function and strengthen neural connections in the brain.

It is important to note that while cognitive stimulation and brain training can be helpful in reducing the risk of developing dementia, they are just one part of a comprehensive approach to brain health. Other factors, such as a healthy diet, getting enough sleep, and managing stress, are also important for maintaining cognitive function.

In conclusion, cognitive stimulation and brain training are effective ways to help reduce the risk of developing dementia and improve overall brain health. By engaging in activities such as playing games and puzzles, reading and learning, staying socially active, exercising, and trying brain training exercises, individuals can promote cognitive function and maintain a healthy brain as they age.

The role of diet and nutrition in brain health

The human brain is a complex organ that requires a variety of nutrients to function properly. As we age, our brain becomes more vulnerable to damage and degeneration, which can result in the development of cognitive impairments, including dementia. However, research has shown that diet and nutrition can play a significant role in reducing the risk of developing dementia and improving brain health.

One of the key factors in maintaining brain health is to consume a diet rich in fruits, vegetables, whole grains, lean protein, and healthy fats. Studies have shown that individuals who follow a Mediterranean-style diet have a lower risk of developing cognitive impairments, including dementia. The Mediterranean diet is high in fruits, vegetables, whole grains, fish, and olive oil, and low in red meat, sugar, and saturated fats. This diet is rich in antioxidants, which help to protect the brain from damage caused by free radicals.

In addition to consuming a healthy diet, it is also important to avoid consuming foods and beverages that are high in sugar, salt, and saturated fats. These foods can lead to inflammation, which can damage brain cells and increase the risk of developing dementia. Processed and packaged foods should also be avoided, as they are often high in unhealthy fats and preservatives.

Another important factor in maintaining brain health is staying hydrated. Dehydration can lead to fatigue, headaches, and poor cognitive function. Drinking plenty of water throughout the day can help to keep the brain hydrated and functioning properly. Consuming foods that are high in water content, such as fruits and vegetables, can also help to keep the body hydrated.

Several nutrients have been shown to be particularly beneficial for brain health. These include omega-3 fatty acids, B vitamins, vitamin D, and antioxidants such as vitamin C and E. Omega-3 fatty acids are found in fish, nuts, and seeds and have been shown to reduce inflammation and improve brain function. B vitamins, particularly vitamin B12, are important for maintaining healthy brain cells and preventing cognitive decline. Vitamin D is essential for brain health, and studies have shown that low levels of vitamin D are associated with an increased risk of developing dementia. Antioxidants such as vitamin C and E are important for protecting the brain from damage caused by free radicals.

In addition to consuming a healthy diet, engaging in regular physical activity is also important for maintaining brain health. Exercise has been shown to improve cognitive function and reduce the risk of developing dementia. Studies have shown that regular physical activity can help to improve memory, attention, and decision-making abilities. Exercise also helps to reduce stress and improve mood, which can have a positive impact on brain health.

Other lifestyle factors that can help to maintain brain health include getting enough sleep, managing stress, and engaging in mentally stimulating activities. Getting enough sleep is essential for allowing the brain to rest and recharge. Chronic stress can lead to inflammation, which can damage brain cells and increase the risk of developing dementia. Engaging in mentally stimulating activities such as reading, playing games, and learning new skills can help to improve cognitive function and reduce the risk of cognitive decline.

In conclusion, diet and nutrition play a critical role in maintaining brain health and reducing the risk of developing dementia. Consuming a diet rich in fruits, vegetables, whole grains, lean protein, and healthy fats can provide the brain with the nutrients it needs to function properly. In addition to diet, staying hydrated, engaging in regular physical activity, getting enough sleep, managing stress, and engaging in mentally stimulating activities can also help to maintain brain health. By adopting healthy lifestyle habits, individuals can reduce their risk of cognitive decline and maintain their cognitive function well into old age.

Chapter Twenty-Three

Technology and Dementia Care

Dementia is a condition that affects millions of people around the world, and the number of those affected is projected to increase in the coming years. While there is currently no cure for dementia, there are many technologies that have been developed to help individuals with dementia and their caregivers manage the condition. Below we will we will explore the role of technology in dementia care, including its benefits and potential drawbacks.

One of the most significant benefits of technology in dementia care is its ability to assist with memory loss. Memory loss is a common symptom of dementia, and it can be challenging for individuals with the condition to remember important information, such as their daily routines, medication schedules, and the names of loved ones. Technology, however, can provide memory aids and reminders that can help individuals with dementia maintain their independence and quality of life.

One example of such technology is the use of electronic calendars and reminder systems. These tools can be programmed to send reminders to individuals with dementia about appointments, medication schedules, and other important events. Additionally, they can be customized to suit the individual's needs and preferences, such as the type of reminder message, the frequency of reminders, and the method of delivery (e.g., visual, auditory).

Another significant benefit of technology in dementia care is its ability to improve communication and social interaction. Communication difficulties are common in individuals with dementia, which can lead to feelings of isolation and loneliness. However, technology such as video conferencing tools and social media platforms can facilitate communication with loved ones and other members of the community, helping individuals with dementia maintain social connections and reduce feelings of loneliness.

For example, video conferencing tools such as Zoom and Skype can allow individuals with dementia to connect with family members and friends who may live far away or be unable to visit in person. Social media platforms such as Facebook and Twitter can also facilitate communication and social interaction, allowing individuals with dementia to share their thoughts and experiences with a wider audience and engage in online communities.

While technology has many benefits for dementia care, there are also potential drawbacks that should be considered. One potential drawback is the cost of technology, which may be prohibitive for some individuals and families. Additionally, some individuals with dementia may find technology challenging to use or may be resistant to its use due to a lack of familiarity or discomfort with technology.

Another potential drawback is the risk of overreliance on technology, which may lead to a decrease in face-to-face interaction and social support. While technology can provide important support and assistance, it cannot replace the benefits of human interaction and social support. Therefore, it is important to strike a balance between the use of technology and other forms of support and engagement.

In conclusion, technology has become an increasingly important tool in dementia care, providing memory aids, communication tools, and other forms of support for individuals with dementia and their caregivers. While technology has many benefits, it is important to consider the potential drawbacks and to use it in conjunction with other forms of support and engagement to ensure the best possible outcomes for individuals with dementia. By doing so, we can improve the quality of life for individuals with dementia and their families and help to address the growing challenge of this condition.

Assistive devices and monitoring systems

Assistive devices and monitoring systems have become increasingly important in dementia care. These technologies can help people with dementia maintain their independence, monitor their health, and keep them safe. Additionally, assistive devices and monitoring systems can help caregivers provide better care and reduce the stress associated with caregiving.

One of the most common assistive devices used in dementia care is a GPS tracker. This device can be worn as a bracelet or attached to a piece of clothing and allows caregivers to track the location of their loved one with dementia. This is particularly helpful for those who tend to wander, a common behavior in people with dementia. GPS trackers can help reduce the risk of getting lost, and can provide peace of mind for both the person with dementia and their caregivers.

Another assistive device is a medication dispenser. This device can help people with dementia remember to take their medication at the correct time. The dispenser can be pre-filled by a caregiver or healthcare professional, and will dispense the correct medication at the correct time. This is particularly helpful for those with memory problems, who may forget to take their medication, or take it multiple times by accident.

Monitoring systems are also becoming increasingly popular in dementia care. These systems can monitor a person's activity, sleep patterns, and health. For example, a monitoring system can detect if a person with dementia has fallen, or if they have not moved for an extended period of time. This information can then be relayed to a caregiver, who can take appropriate action.

In addition to assistive devices and monitoring systems, technology is also being used to provide cognitive stimulation for people with dementia. Apps and games designed specifically for people with dementia can help improve memory, cognitive function, and overall brain health. These apps can be used independently by the person with dementia, or with the assistance of a caregiver.

While assistive devices and monitoring systems can be incredibly helpful in dementia care, it is important to note that they should not replace the human touch. Caregivers should continue to provide emotional support, engage in meaningful activities with their loved one, and ensure their physical needs are met. Assistive devices and monitoring systems should be used as a tool to supplement care, not replace it.

There are also some potential drawbacks to the use of assistive devices and monitoring systems. One concern is the potential loss of privacy and independence for the person with dementia. The constant monitoring and use of assistive devices can make a person with dementia feel like they are being watched or controlled. Additionally, the cost of some of these devices and systems can be a barrier for some families.

In conclusion, assistive devices and monitoring systems can play an important role in dementia care. They can help people with dementia maintain their independence, keep them safe, and provide peace of mind for caregivers. However, it is important to use these technologies as a supplement to human care, and to be aware of potential privacy concerns. By carefully considering the use of these devices and systems, caregivers can provide better care for their loved ones with dementia.

Telehealth and remote care options

Dementia is a progressive disease that can severely impact an individual's ability to perform daily activities, communicate effectively, and maintain their independence. As the number of people with dementia continues to rise, there is a growing need for effective and accessible care options, including telehealth and remote care. Below we will we will explore the benefits and challenges of telehealth and remote care options for dementia patients.

Telehealth, also known as telemedicine, refers to the use of technology to provide medical care and services remotely. This can include video conferencing, remote monitoring, and other forms of digital communication. Telehealth has become increasingly popular in recent years, and has been shown to improve access to care, reduce healthcare costs, and improve patient outcomes. For dementia patients, telehealth can offer numerous benefits.

One of the primary benefits of telehealth for dementia patients is improved access to care. Many dementia patients live in rural or remote areas, where access to specialized care can be limited. Telehealth can allow patients to connect with healthcare professionals, even if they are located far away. This can help to ensure that patients receive timely and appropriate care, which can improve their quality of life and overall health.

Another benefit of telehealth for dementia patients is increased convenience. Many dementia patients experience challenges with transportation and mobility, which can make it difficult to attend appointments in person. Telehealth can eliminate the need for patients to travel to appointments, which can help to reduce stress and improve their overall experience.

Telehealth can also offer dementia patients greater independence and autonomy. By providing remote care options, patients can continue to live in their own homes and communities for longer periods of time. This can help to improve their overall quality of life, and can reduce the burden on caregivers and family members.

Despite these benefits, there are also challenges associated with telehealth and remote care options for dementia patients. One of the primary challenges is ensuring that patients receive the same level of care as they would in-person. This can be especially challenging for patients with complex needs, such as those with advanced dementia.

Another challenge is ensuring that patients are able to effectively communicate with healthcare professionals through remote means. Dementia patients may experience difficulty with speech and language, which can make it challenging to communicate through video conferencing or other digital means. Additionally, patients with hearing or vision impairments may require specialized accommodations in order to effectively communicate with healthcare professionals.

There are also concerns about privacy and security when it comes to telehealth and remote care options for dementia patients. As with any form of digital communication, there is a risk of data breaches or other security issues. It is important to ensure that patient information is protected and secure when using telehealth or remote care options.

Despite these challenges, the use of telehealth and remote care options for dementia patients is growing. In recent years, there has been a significant increase in the use of telehealth, and this trend is expected to continue. As technology continues to advance, there will likely be new and innovative ways to provide remote care to dementia patients.

In conclusion, telehealth and remote care options can offer numerous benefits for dementia patients, including improved access to care, increased convenience, and greater independence and autonomy. While there are challenges associated with these options, they have the potential to significantly improve the lives of dementia patients and their families. As healthcare providers continue to explore new and innovative ways to deliver care, it is important to consider the benefits and challenges of telehealth and remote care options for dementia patients.

Innovative technological advancements in dementia care

In recent years, technological advancements have significantly impacted the field of dementia care. New tools and devices have emerged to aid individuals living with dementia and their caregivers in managing symptoms and improving overall quality of life. These technological advancements are particularly important as the number of people living with dementia is expected to increase globally.

One significant area of technological innovation in dementia care is assistive devices. These devices are designed to aid individuals with dementia in performing activities of daily living and maintaining independence for as long as possible. Examples of assistive devices include personal alarm systems, which can alert caregivers or emergency services in the event of a fall or other emergency, and medication reminders, which can help individuals with dementia remember to take their medications on time.

Another area of innovation in dementia care is the development of monitoring systems. These systems use sensors to monitor an individual's movements and behavior, providing caregivers with real-time information about their loved one's activities. This information can be used to identify changes in behavior that may indicate a decline in cognitive or physical health. Monitoring systems can also be used to improve safety, by alerting caregivers if an individual with dementia has wandered outside of a designated area or if there is a risk of falls.

Telehealth and remote care options have also emerged as important tools in dementia care. These technologies allow individuals with dementia to receive medical care and support from the comfort of their own homes. Telehealth platforms can be used to conduct virtual appointments with healthcare professionals, while remote care options such as video monitoring can allow caregivers to remotely monitor their loved one's health and well-being.

Innovative technologies are also being developed to improve communication and social engagement for individuals with dementia. For example, digital devices such as tablets and smartphones can be used to facilitate video calls with friends and family members, as well as to access social media and other online platforms. Virtual reality technology is also being explored as a tool for improving social engagement and reducing feelings of isolation among individuals with dementia.

One particularly promising area of technological innovation in dementia care is the use of artificial intelligence (AI) and machine learning. These technologies have the potential to revolutionize dementia care by providing more accurate and personalized diagnoses and treatment recommendations. AI and machine learning algorithms can analyze large amounts of data to identify patterns and predict outcomes, which can help healthcare professionals make more informed decisions about treatment and care.

In addition to these technological advancements, there is also growing interest in the use of robots in dementia care. Robots can be programmed to provide assistance with tasks such as bathing and dressing, and they can also be used to provide social engagement and emotional support for individuals with dementia.

Overall, the use of technology in dementia care has the potential to significantly improve the lives of individuals with dementia and their caregivers. These technological advancements can help individuals with dementia maintain independence and improve overall quality of life, while also providing caregivers with valuable support and resources. As technology continues to advance, it is likely that even more innovative tools and devices will emerge to aid in the care of individuals with dementia.

Chapter Twenty-Four

Education and Training for Professionals

Dementia is a complex and challenging condition that affects millions of people worldwide. It can be difficult for healthcare professionals to navigate the complexities of dementia care, which is why education and training are critical components of dementia care. Education and training can help professionals understand the unique needs of people with dementia, develop effective care plans, and provide compassionate and competent care.

One of the key aspects of education and training for dementia care is understanding the nature of the disease. Dementia is a progressive condition that affects memory, cognition, and behavior. There are different types of dementia, including Alzheimer's disease, vascular dementia, Lewy body dementia, and frontotemporal dementia. Each type of dementia has its unique symptoms, causes, and treatment options. Understanding these differences is critical for developing effective care plans and providing appropriate care.

Another important aspect of education and training for dementia care is understanding the challenges faced by people with dementia and their families. Dementia can be a challenging and isolating condition that can have a significant impact on a person's quality of life. It is essential that healthcare professionals understand the challenges faced by people with dementia and their families so they can provide compassionate and empathetic care.

One of the most significant challenges faced by people with dementia is communication. As the disease progresses, it can become increasingly difficult for people with dementia to communicate effectively. This can lead to frustration, isolation, and social withdrawal. Healthcare professionals need to be trained in effective communication techniques, such as using simple and clear language, avoiding abstract concepts, and using visual aids, to help people with dementia communicate their needs and wishes effectively.

Another critical component of education and training for dementia care is developing care plans that are tailored to the unique needs of each person with dementia. Care plans should take into account the person's individual needs, preferences, and abilities. They should also be flexible enough to adapt to changes in the person's condition. Developing effective care plans requires a comprehensive understanding of the person's medical history, cognitive abilities, and daily routines.

Training in dementia care should also include training in behavioral management techniques. People with dementia may exhibit challenging behaviors such as agitation, aggression, and wandering. Healthcare professionals need to be trained in effective behavioral management techniques, such as diversional therapy, validation therapy, and behavioral interventions, to manage these behaviors effectively.

Finally, education and training in dementia care should also focus on the importance of providing support to families and caregivers. Caring for a loved one with dementia can be emotionally and physically exhausting, and caregivers may need support and guidance to manage the challenges of caregiving effectively. Healthcare professionals need to be trained in providing emotional support and practical advice to families and caregivers to ensure they are well-equipped to provide care.

In conclusion, education and training for dementia care are essential components of providing high-quality care to people with dementia. It is essential that healthcare professionals understand the unique needs of people with dementia, develop effective care plans, and provide compassionate and competent care. By investing in education and training for dementia care, healthcare professionals can improve the quality of life for people with dementia and their families, reduce caregiver burden, and ultimately improve the overall health outcomes for people with dementia.

Dementia care training for healthcare providers

Dementia is a chronic and progressive neurological condition that can have a significant impact on the physical, emotional, and social well-being of individuals affected by it. As the number of individuals diagnosed with dementia continues to rise, there is an increasing need for healthcare providers to have specialized training in dementia care. Below we will discuss the importance of dementia care training for healthcare providers and the different types of training available.

Dementia care training is crucial for healthcare providers as it equips them with the knowledge and skills needed to provide quality care for individuals with dementia. Healthcare providers need to understand the unique challenges that individuals with dementia face, such as memory loss, difficulty with communication, and behavioral changes. They also need to be able to provide individualized care that takes into account the individual's specific needs and preferences.

One of the most significant benefits of dementia care training is that it can improve the quality of care that individuals with dementia receive. Healthcare providers who receive specialized training are better equipped to provide care that is tailored to the needs of the individual. They can also help individuals with dementia maintain their independence and improve their overall quality of life.

Another benefit of dementia care training is that it can reduce the burden on caregivers. Healthcare providers who have received specialized training can work collaboratively with caregivers to provide comprehensive care for individuals with dementia. This can help to reduce caregiver stress and burnout, which can have a significant impact on their own health and well-being.

There are several different types of dementia care training available for healthcare providers. One type of training is basic dementia awareness training, which provides an overview of the different types of dementia and the common symptoms associated with the condition. This type of training is useful for healthcare providers who are new to working with individuals with dementia.

Another type of training is person-centered care training, which focuses on providing care that is tailored to the individual's specific needs and preferences. This type of training is particularly important for healthcare providers who work in long-term care settings, where individuals with dementia may have complex care needs.

Communication training is also an essential component of dementia care training. Healthcare providers need to be able to communicate effectively with individuals with dementia, as they may have difficulty with language and communication. Communication training can help healthcare providers to understand how to communicate with individuals with dementia in a way that is clear and effective.

Training in behavioral management is also important for healthcare providers working with individuals with dementia. Behavioral changes are common in individuals with dementia and can be challenging to manage.

Healthcare providers need to understand how to identify and manage these behaviors effectively.

In addition to these types of training, there are also specialized training programs available for healthcare providers who work in specific settings, such as home care or hospice care. These programs provide training that is tailored to the specific needs of the setting and the individuals being cared for.

In conclusion, dementia care training is essential for healthcare providers who work with individuals with dementia. It equips healthcare providers with the knowledge and skills needed to provide quality care that is tailored to the individual's specific needs and preferences. There are several different types of dementia care training available, including basic dementia awareness training, person-centered care training, communication training, and behavioral management training. Healthcare providers who have received specialized dementia care training can provide comprehensive care that improves the quality of life for individuals with dementia and reduces the burden on caregivers.

Specialized certifications and continuing education

As the number of individuals living with dementia continues to rise, there is a growing need for specialized healthcare professionals who are knowledgeable and skilled in providing quality dementia care. Specialized certifications and continuing education opportunities play an essential role in ensuring healthcare professionals are adequately equipped to provide the best possible care for individuals living with dementia.

One such certification is the Certified Dementia Practitioner (CDP) credential offered by the National Council of Certified Dementia Practitioners (NCCDP). This certification program is designed to provide healthcare professionals with in-depth knowledge of dementia and effective strategies for providing care to individuals living with the condition. The program covers a broad range of topics, including communication techniques, behavior management, activities for individuals with dementia, and end-of-life care.

Continuing education opportunities, such as conferences and workshops, can also be an invaluable resource for healthcare professionals seeking to expand their knowledge and skills in dementia care. The Alzheimer's Association, for example, offers a range of educational programs and events, including the annual International Conference on Alzheimer's Disease and Dementia. These programs provide healthcare professionals with access to the latest research and best practices in dementia care.

In addition to specialized certifications and continuing education opportunities, healthcare organizations can also implement ongoing training and support programs for staff members. These programs can help ensure that staff members are consistently providing high-quality care to individuals living with dementia.

One example of such a program is the Dementia Care Specialist Program offered by the HealthCare Interactive (HCI) organization. This program provides healthcare organizations with a comprehensive training and support system designed to enhance staff members' knowledge and skills in dementia care. The program includes an online training course, ongoing support and coaching from HCI staff members, and access to a variety of resources and tools.

The benefits of specialized certifications and continuing education opportunities in dementia care are numerous. For healthcare professionals, these programs provide a means of acquiring the knowledge and skills necessary to provide quality care to individuals living with dementia. They also demonstrate a commitment to ongoing professional development and a desire to provide the best possible care to patients.

For individuals living with dementia and their families, specialized certifications and ongoing training programs can provide assurance that they are receiving care from knowledgeable and skilled professionals who are dedicated to providing high-quality care. This can lead to increased trust and confidence in the healthcare system and may ultimately improve health outcomes for individuals living with dementia.

Overall, specialized certifications and continuing education opportunities are essential components of dementia care. They provide healthcare professionals with the knowledge and skills necessary to provide quality care to individuals living with the condition, and they can also improve outcomes for patients and their families. As the need for specialized dementia care continues to grow, it is crucial that healthcare organizations prioritize ongoing training and professional development for their staff members to ensure the best possible outcomes for all individuals affected by dementia.

Best practices in dementia care

Dementia is a complex and challenging condition that affects millions of people worldwide. As the number of individuals living with dementia continues to grow, it is crucial to develop and implement best practices in dementia care. Effective care can enhance quality of life, promote independence and autonomy, and provide support to both individuals with dementia and their families.

One of the key best practices in dementia care is person-centered care. This approach prioritizes the individual's unique needs, preferences, and strengths, and ensures that they are involved in decision-making as much as possible. It is important to recognize that every person with dementia is unique, with their own life experiences, beliefs, and values. By taking a person-centered approach, caregivers can better understand and meet the needs of each individual they serve.

Communication is also critical in dementia care. Communication challenges are common in individuals with dementia, and caregivers must be trained to use effective communication techniques to support these individuals. These techniques may include using nonverbal cues, speaking slowly and clearly, and using positive language. Additionally, caregivers must be prepared to handle communication challenges that may arise due to cultural differences, hearing or vision impairments, or other factors.

Another best practice in dementia care is to promote a safe and supportive environment. This may include modifying the physical environment to reduce hazards and increase comfort, as well as providing emotional support to individuals with dementia and their families. Caregivers must also be trained to recognize and respond to potential safety risks, such as wandering or falls.

There are several evidence-based interventions that have been shown to be effective in supporting individuals with dementia. These interventions may include cognitive stimulation therapy, reminiscence therapy, and behavioral interventions. Additionally, physical exercise and other forms of physical activity have been found to improve cognitive function, physical health, and overall quality of life in individuals with dementia.

Effective dementia care also requires collaboration and coordination among healthcare providers, family members, and other caregivers. Interdisciplinary care teams may include physicians, nurses, social workers, and other healthcare professionals who work together to develop and implement a care plan that meets the individual's unique needs.

Finally, ongoing education and training are critical in ensuring that caregivers are equipped with the knowledge and skills needed to provide effective dementia care. This includes initial training for new caregivers, as well as ongoing professional development opportunities for experienced caregivers. Training may include topics such as communication techniques, person-centered care, and evidence-based interventions.

In conclusion, dementia care is a complex and challenging field that requires a person-centered approach, effective communication, a safe and supportive environment, evidence-based interventions, interdisciplinary care, and ongoing education and training for caregivers. By implementing best practices in dementia care, individuals with dementia can receive the support they need to maintain their quality of life and maximize their independence and autonomy.

Chapter Twenty-Five

Resources and Support Networks

Dementia can be an overwhelming and isolating experience for both individuals living with the condition and their loved ones. Fortunately, there are many resources and support networks available to help navigate the challenges of dementia and improve overall quality of life.

One important resource for those living with dementia and their families is support groups. These groups offer a safe and non-judgmental space to share experiences and learn from others going through similar challenges. Support groups can be found through local community organizations, senior centers, or online forums. They can be especially beneficial for caregivers who may feel isolated or overwhelmed by their responsibilities.

Another resource for dementia care is counseling or therapy. This can be helpful for individuals living with dementia who may be experiencing anxiety, depression, or other emotional challenges related to their condition. Therapy can also be helpful for caregivers who may be experiencing stress, burnout, or grief.

In addition to support groups and counseling, there are many online resources available for those impacted by dementia. The Alzheimer's Association, for example, offers a wealth of information on their website, including educational materials, caregiver resources, and information about clinical trials. Other organizations, such as the Lewy Body Dementia Association or the Association for Frontotemporal Degeneration, offer support and resources for those impacted by specific types of dementia.

There are also many technological resources available for those living with dementia and their families. For example, there are devices that can help with medication management or remind individuals of important appointments or tasks. There are also GPS tracking devices that can help locate individuals who may wander or become lost.

Furthermore, there are several government programs that offer resources and support for those living with dementia. Medicare, for example, offers coverage for certain dementia-related services, such as cognitive assessments and counseling. Medicaid may also offer financial assistance for long-term care services. Additionally, the Administration on Aging offers programs and services that support individuals with dementia and their caregivers.

One often-overlooked resource for dementia care is community organizations and volunteers. Many communities have organizations or volunteers who can provide assistance with tasks such as transportation, grocery shopping, or meal preparation. This can be especially helpful for individuals living with dementia who may have difficulty completing these tasks on their own.

It is also important to recognize the importance of legal and financial planning in dementia care. Individuals with dementia and their families should work with an attorney to create legal documents such as power of attorney or advance directives. This can help ensure that their wishes are carried out in the event of incapacity. Financial planning is also important to ensure that individuals with dementia have access to the resources they need for long-term care.

Finally, it is important to recognize that dementia care is not a one-size-fits-all approach. Different individuals may require different types of support and resources. It is important to work with healthcare providers, social workers, and other professionals to develop a personalized care plan that meets the unique needs of each individual impacted by dementia.

In conclusion, there are many resources and support networks available for those impacted by dementia. These resources can help improve overall quality of life for individuals with dementia and their families. It is important to take advantage of these resources and to work with healthcare providers and other professionals to develop a personalized care plan. By doing so, individuals impacted by dementia can receive the care and support they need to live full and meaningful lives.

National and international dementia organizations

Dementia is a global health concern that affects millions of individuals worldwide. As a result, there are numerous national and international organizations dedicated to improving dementia care, supporting individuals living with dementia and their families, and funding research to better understand the condition. Below we will we will discuss some of the major national and international dementia organizations and the work they do.

One of the largest international dementia organizations is Alzheimer's Disease International (ADI). ADI was founded in 1984 and is now the global umbrella organization for over 100 Alzheimer's and dementia associations worldwide. The organization works to raise awareness about dementia, promote early diagnosis and intervention, and advocate for better dementia care and support services. ADI also hosts an annual conference, the Alzheimer's Disease International Conference, which brings together researchers, healthcare professionals, and individuals living with dementia and their families from around the world to share the latest research and best practices in dementia care.

Another major international organization is the World Dementia Council (WDC). The WDC was established in 2013 as a response to the global dementia crisis. Its mission is to provide leadership and guidance to international efforts to combat dementia, including accelerating research, developing innovative care models, and promoting best practices in dementia care. The WDC consists of international leaders in dementia research, policy, and advocacy, including government officials, healthcare professionals, and individuals living with dementia and their families.

In the United States, one of the largest national dementia organizations is the Alzheimer's Association. The Alzheimer's Association is the largest nonprofit organization dedicated to Alzheimer's and dementia care, support, and research. The organization provides a range of services and resources, including a national helpline, support groups, educational materials, and advocacy initiatives. The Alzheimer's Association also funds research aimed at better understanding the causes and potential treatments for dementia.

Another major national organization is the National Institute on Aging (NIA), which is part of the National Institutes of Health (NIH). The NIA is the primary federal agency for conducting and funding research on aging and age-related conditions, including dementia. The organization funds research aimed at better understanding the biology of aging and age-related diseases, developing new treatments for dementia, and improving dementia care and support services. The NIA also provides educational materials and resources for healthcare professionals and individuals living with dementia and their families.

In the United Kingdom, one of the largest national dementia organizations is the Alzheimer's Society. The Alzheimer's Society provides a range of services and resources, including information and advice, support groups, and dementia care training for healthcare professionals. The organization also funds research into the causes and potential treatments for dementia and advocates for better dementia care and support services in the UK.

Another major national organization in the UK is Dementia UK. Dementia UK provides specialist dementia support and advice through its Admiral Nurse service. Admiral Nurses are specialist dementia nurses who provide one-to-one support and advice for individuals living with dementia and their families. The organization also funds research into dementia care and works to raise awareness about dementia and reduce the stigma associated with the condition.

In Canada, one of the largest national dementia organizations is the Alzheimer Society of Canada. The Alzheimer Society of Canada provides a range of services and resources, including a national helpline, support groups, and educational materials. The organization also funds research into the causes and potential treatments for dementia and advocates for better dementia care and support services in Canada.

Another major national organization in Canada is the Centre for Aging and Brain Health Innovation (CABHI). CABHI is a national organization that supports the development and implementation of innovative aging and brain health solutions, including technology-based solutions for dementia care. The organization provides funding for research and development projects and works to bring together researchers, healthcare professionals, and industry partners to develop and implement innovative solutions for dementia care.

Online forums and support groups

Online forums and support groups are becoming increasingly popular among people living with dementia, caregivers, and family members seeking emotional support, advice, and information. These online platforms have revolutionized the way we communicate and share information, and have the potential to provide significant benefits to those impacted by dementia.

One of the main advantages of online forums and support groups is the ability to connect with others who are experiencing similar challenges. This can be especially helpful for individuals with dementia who may feel isolated and lonely due to their condition. Caregivers can also benefit from these online communities as they can connect with others who are going through similar experiences, and gain insight into different care strategies and coping mechanisms.

Another advantage of online support groups is the access to information and resources that they provide. These forums often have knowledgeable members who can share their experiences and provide valuable advice on navigating the various challenges associated with dementia. Members can also share links to relevant websites, articles, and research studies, providing a wealth of information at the click of a button.

Online support groups can be particularly beneficial for people who live in rural or remote areas where access to support services may be limited. These individuals may find it challenging to attend in-person support groups due to distance or mobility issues, but online forums can provide a sense of community and support without the need to travel.

While there are many benefits to online forums and support groups, it is important to exercise caution and be mindful of potential risks. The anonymity of the internet means that not everyone on these forums has good intentions, and misinformation and scams can be prevalent. It is important to verify the accuracy of any information obtained online and to be wary of any unsolicited messages or requests for personal information.

There are many different online forums and support groups available for people living with dementia, their caregivers, and families. The Alzheimer's Association offers a 24/7 online community where members can share their experiences, ask questions, and receive support. The Dementia Support Group on Facebook is another popular forum where members can connect with others impacted by dementia and share information and resources. There are also many other online support groups dedicated to specific types of dementia, such as Lewy body dementia and frontotemporal dementia.

In addition to online forums and support groups, there are also many resources available to help individuals living with dementia and their caregivers. The Alzheimer's Association offers a wealth of information on their website, including resources on dementia care, legal and financial planning, and tips for living with dementia. The National Institute on Aging also offers a variety of resources on their website, including information on clinical trials and treatment options.

In conclusion, online forums and support groups can provide valuable support, information, and resources to individuals living with dementia, their caregivers, and families. While caution should be exercised, the benefits of these online communities can be significant, especially for those who may not have access to in-person support services. It is important to stay informed and connected to others during the journey with dementia, and online support groups can be a great tool for achieving this.

Educational materials and resources for families and caregivers

Dementia is a complex disease that can have a significant impact on both the individual with the condition and their caregivers. It is a progressive disorder that affects the brain, leading to a decline in cognitive function, memory loss, and difficulties with everyday activities. Providing care for someone with dementia can be challenging and stressful, and caregivers often require resources and support to help them provide the best care possible. Educational materials and resources for families and caregivers can provide valuable information and support, helping caregivers to better understand the disease and the needs of those living with dementia.

One of the most important aspects of providing care for someone with dementia is understanding the disease itself. Educational materials can provide caregivers with information about the causes of dementia, the various types of dementia, and the symptoms that can be associated with the disease. Understanding these aspects of dementia can help caregivers to better anticipate and manage the needs of their loved ones. For example, caregivers may learn about how to recognize signs of distress or agitation in individuals with dementia, and how to use calming techniques to help manage these symptoms.

Educational materials can also provide caregivers with information about how to communicate effectively with individuals with dementia. As the disease progresses, communication can become increasingly difficult, and individuals with dementia may experience difficulty expressing themselves or understanding others. Caregivers can learn techniques for effective communication, such as using simple language, using visual aids, and maintaining eye contact. These strategies can help to reduce confusion and frustration for both the caregiver and the individual with dementia.

Caregivers can also benefit from educational materials that provide information about strategies for managing behavioral symptoms associated with dementia, such as agitation, aggression, and wandering. These materials can offer tips and advice on how to handle difficult behaviors in a calm and effective manner, as well as strategies for preventing challenging behaviors from occurring in the first place. Additionally, caregivers can learn about the use of medication and other interventions that may be helpful in managing these symptoms.

Another important aspect of dementia care is managing daily activities and routines. Educational materials can provide caregivers with guidance on how to structure daily activities in a way that is both safe and stimulating for individuals with dementia. This may involve creating a routine for meals, bathing, and other daily tasks, as well as engaging individuals with dementia in activities that promote social interaction and cognitive stimulation.

Finally, educational materials can provide caregivers with information about support services and resources that are available in their community. This may include local support groups, respite care services, and resources for financial assistance. Caregivers can learn about the availability of these resources, how to access them, and how they can be of benefit to both themselves and their loved ones with dementia.

In conclusion, providing care for someone with dementia can be challenging and stressful. Educational materials and resources for families and caregivers can provide valuable information and support, helping caregivers to better understand the disease and the needs of those living with dementia. By providing caregivers with information about the disease, effective communication strategies, management of behavioral symptoms, daily activities and routines, and available support services, caregivers can better equip themselves to provide the best possible care for their loved ones with dementia.

Chapter Twenty-Six

Navigating the Healthcare System

Navigating the healthcare system can be a complex and overwhelming process for anyone, but it can be especially challenging for individuals with dementia and their caregivers. Dementia is a progressive brain disorder that affects cognitive abilities, such as memory, thinking, and reasoning. As the disease progresses, individuals with dementia may require more specialized care and support, including navigating the healthcare system.

One of the key challenges that individuals with dementia and their caregivers face when navigating the healthcare system is ensuring that they receive appropriate and timely care. This can be especially difficult for those who are not familiar with the healthcare system or who have limited resources. Additionally, communication difficulties may arise due to the cognitive impairment associated with dementia, making it difficult for individuals to express their needs and for healthcare providers to understand them.

One way to overcome these challenges is to establish a relationship with a primary care physician who is familiar with dementia and its associated care needs. This can help ensure that individuals with dementia receive appropriate and timely care, and can also help prevent unnecessary hospitalizations or emergency room visits. Additionally, it may be helpful to engage the services of a dementia care specialist or geriatrician, who has specialized training in the care of older adults with dementia.

Another important aspect of navigating the healthcare system for individuals with dementia is advocating for their needs and ensuring that they are receiving appropriate care. This may involve advocating for additional resources or support services, such as home health aides or respite care, or advocating for appropriate medications or treatments. It may also involve working with healthcare providers to ensure that they understand the unique needs of individuals with dementia, and that they are taking steps to address these needs.

It is also important for individuals with dementia and their caregivers to be informed about the various resources and support services available to them. This may include community-based programs, such as support groups or adult day care centers, as well as government-funded programs, such as Medicare and Medicaid. Additionally, there are a variety of non-profit organizations that provide support and education to individuals with dementia and their caregivers, such as the Alzheimer's Association and the Lewy Body Dementia Association.

One of the challenges of navigating the healthcare system for individuals with dementia is the potential for misdiagnosis or inappropriate treatment. Due to the complexity of the disease and the difficulty in diagnosing dementia, it is important for individuals and their caregivers to seek out the services of healthcare providers who have experience and expertise in the care of individuals with dementia. Additionally, it may be helpful to seek out second opinions or to consult with multiple healthcare providers to ensure that the individual with dementia is receiving appropriate care.

Finally, it is important for individuals with dementia and their caregivers to have a plan in place for future care needs. This may involve establishing a power of attorney or advance directive, or making decisions about end-of-life care. By having a plan in place, individuals and their caregivers can ensure that their wishes are being respected and that they are receiving appropriate care, even if they are unable to make decisions for themselves.

In conclusion, navigating the healthcare system can be a complex and challenging process for individuals with dementia and their caregivers. However, by establishing a relationship with a primary care physician or dementia care specialist, advocating for their needs, accessing resources and support services, seeking out appropriate diagnosis and treatment, and planning for future care needs, individuals with dementia and their caregivers can ensure that they are receiving appropriate and timely care. It is important for individuals and their caregivers to be informed about their options and to seek out the support and resources they need to successfully navigate the healthcare system.

Coordinating care among healthcare providers

As dementia progresses, patients often require care from multiple healthcare providers, including primary care physicians, specialists, and support staff. Coordinating care among these various providers can be challenging, but it is crucial for ensuring that patients receive high-quality, integrated care. Below we will we will discuss the importance of coordinating care among healthcare providers for individuals with dementia.

Dementia is a complex disease that affects multiple areas of the brain, resulting in a wide range of symptoms, including memory loss, confusion, and difficulty with communication and daily activities. As the disease progresses, patients often require care from multiple healthcare providers, including neurologists, geriatricians, psychiatrists, and social workers. These providers may work in different locations and may not have access to all of the patient's medical records, making it difficult to ensure that the patient receives consistent and appropriate care.

Coordinating care among healthcare providers is essential for individuals with dementia, as it helps ensure that all of their medical and social needs are met. This involves a team-based approach to care, with each provider contributing their expertise to ensure that the patient receives comprehensive care. For example, a primary care physician may oversee the patient's overall care, while a neurologist may focus on managing symptoms related to cognitive decline.

To coordinate care effectively, healthcare providers must communicate with each other regularly and share information about the patient's health status, medications, and care plans. This can be challenging, as providers may have different schedules and work in different locations. To overcome these barriers, some healthcare systems have implemented electronic health records (EHRs) that allow providers to access patient records from any location. Additionally, some healthcare systems have implemented care coordination teams that help manage communication and ensure that all providers are aware of changes in the patient's health status.

In addition to coordinating care among healthcare providers, it is also essential to involve family members and other caregivers in the care process. Family members and caregivers can provide valuable information about the patient's health status and help ensure that the patient receives consistent care. They can also help with tasks such as medication management, transportation, and daily activities.

One approach to involving family members and caregivers in the care process is to implement a care team model. In this model, a designated care coordinator works with the patient and their family members to develop a care plan that meets the patient's needs. The care coordinator then works with healthcare providers and other members of the care team to implement the care plan and ensure that everyone is aware of changes in the patient's health status.

In addition to the care team model, there are other tools and resources available to help healthcare providers and caregivers coordinate care for individuals with dementia. For example, some healthcare systems offer caregiver support groups that provide education and emotional support to family members and caregivers. Additionally, there are online resources, such as the Alzheimer's Association and the National Institute on Aging, that provide information and resources for individuals with dementia and their caregivers.

In conclusion, coordinating care among healthcare providers is essential for individuals with dementia. It helps ensure that patients receive comprehensive, integrated care that meets their medical and social needs. To coordinate care effectively, healthcare providers must communicate regularly and share information about the patient's health status, medications, and care plans. Additionally, involving family members and caregivers in the care process can provide valuable information and support. By working together, healthcare providers and caregivers can help ensure that individuals with dementia receive high-quality, coordinated care.

Understanding insurance coverage and benefits

Dementia is a complex and challenging condition that can affect not only the individual diagnosed with it but also their families and caregivers. While there is no cure for dementia, there are various treatments and support services available to help manage the symptoms and improve the quality of life of those affected. However, navigating the healthcare system and understanding insurance coverage and benefits can be overwhelming and confusing for many.

One of the first steps in understanding insurance coverage and benefits is to know what type of insurance plan an individual has. Medicare is a federal health insurance program that covers individuals aged 65 and older or those under 65 with certain disabilities. Medicaid, on the other hand, is a joint federal-state program that provides health insurance for individuals with limited income and resources. Private health insurance plans are also available and may offer more comprehensive coverage than Medicare or Medicaid.

It is important for individuals and their families to understand the specific benefits and limitations of their insurance coverage, as this can vary greatly depending on the plan. Some insurance plans may cover certain types of care, such as home health services, while others may not. It is also important to understand any deductibles, co-payments, or out-of-pocket expenses that may be required.

Navigating the healthcare system can also involve coordinating care among multiple healthcare providers. Dementia care often involves a team of healthcare professionals, including primary care physicians, neurologists, psychiatrists, and social workers. It is important for these professionals to communicate and collaborate to ensure that the individual with dementia receives the most comprehensive and coordinated care possible.

One way to coordinate care among healthcare providers is to designate a primary care physician who can serve as a point of contact and coordinate referrals to other specialists as needed. It is also important to communicate any changes in the individual's condition or medication regimen to all healthcare providers involved in their care.

In addition to healthcare providers, individuals with dementia and their families may also benefit from working with an elder law attorney or financial planner to understand and navigate the legal and financial aspects of dementia care. This may include setting up advance directives, such as a living will or durable power of attorney for healthcare, and managing finances and assets to ensure that the individual with dementia is able to receive the necessary care without depleting their savings.

Finally, it is important for individuals with dementia and their families to be aware of community resources and support networks available to them. These may include local support groups, adult day programs, and respite care services, which can provide a break for caregivers and help individuals with dementia socialize and engage in activities outside the home.

There are also national and international organizations dedicated to supporting individuals with dementia and their families, such as the Alzheimer's Association and the World Dementia Council. These organizations offer educational materials, support networks, and advocacy initiatives to raise awareness and promote research on dementia.

In conclusion, understanding insurance coverage and benefits, coordinating care among healthcare providers, and accessing community resources and support networks can be crucial in navigating the healthcare system and managing the challenges of dementia care. While it can be overwhelming and confusing, there are resources and services available to help individuals with dementia and their families access the care and support they need.

Advocating for the person with dementia

Dementia is a progressive and often debilitating disease that affects an individual's memory, cognitive function, and ability to carry out daily activities. As the disease progresses, individuals with dementia often require increased support and assistance from caregivers and healthcare providers. It is important for individuals with dementia and their families to understand their rights and advocate for their needs throughout the course of the disease.

Advocating for the person with dementia can take many forms. It can involve educating oneself about the disease and its progression, as well as understanding the available resources and support networks. It can also involve being an active participant in the care planning process and communicating one's needs and desires to healthcare providers and caregivers.

One important aspect of advocating for the person with dementia is understanding and asserting their legal rights. This can include ensuring that the person with dementia has access to appropriate medical care and treatment, as well as ensuring that their rights to privacy, dignity, and autonomy are respected. In some cases, legal assistance may be necessary to protect these rights.

It is also important for family members and caregivers to advocate for the person with dementia in healthcare settings. This may involve ensuring that the person receives appropriate care and treatment in hospital or long-term care facilities, as well as advocating for their quality of life and overall well-being. In some cases, family members and caregivers may need to work with healthcare providers to address concerns or advocate for changes in care plans.

In addition to legal and healthcare advocacy, individuals with dementia and their families can also advocate for increased research and funding for dementia care and support. This can involve participating in clinical trials and research studies, as well as supporting advocacy organizations that work to improve dementia care and support for individuals and families affected by the disease.

Another important aspect of advocating for the person with dementia is promoting understanding and awareness of the disease in the broader community. This can involve educating others about the disease and its impact on individuals and families, as well as working to reduce stigma and misconceptions surrounding dementia.

Overall, advocating for the person with dementia requires a multi-faceted approach that includes legal, healthcare, research, and community advocacy. By being informed and proactive, individuals with dementia and their families can ensure that their needs are met and that they receive the highest quality care and support throughout the course of the disease.

Chapter Twenty-Seven

Alternative and Complementary Therapies

Alternative and complementary therapies have become increasingly popular in recent years for managing symptoms and improving quality of life for people with dementia. These therapies include a wide range of interventions that are not typically part of mainstream medical care. While some alternative therapies have shown promise in improving symptoms of dementia, others lack sufficient evidence to support their use.

One alternative therapy that has gained attention in recent years is music therapy. Research has shown that listening to music can stimulate various parts of the brain and can improve mood, reduce agitation, and enhance communication in people with dementia. Music therapy may involve playing musical instruments, singing, or simply listening to music. It can be delivered one-on-one or in a group setting.

Another alternative therapy that has shown promise in managing symptoms of dementia is art therapy. This therapy involves using creative activities, such as painting, drawing, and sculpting, to stimulate the brain and encourage expression. Art therapy has been shown to reduce agitation, improve mood, and enhance cognitive function in people with dementia.

In addition to music and art therapy, other alternative therapies that have shown promise in managing symptoms of dementia include aromatherapy, massage, and acupuncture. Aromatherapy involves using essential oils to enhance mood and reduce anxiety, while massage and acupuncture involve physical manipulation to reduce pain and improve circulation.

While some alternative therapies have shown promise in improving symptoms of dementia, it is important to note that not all alternative therapies are effective or safe. Some alternative therapies may even be harmful, particularly if they are not administered correctly or if they interact with other medications.

It is important to talk with a healthcare provider before starting any alternative therapy for dementia. They can provide guidance on which therapies may be appropriate and safe, and can monitor for any potential side effects or interactions with other medications.

Complementary therapies, on the other hand, are interventions that are used in conjunction with mainstream medical care. These therapies can include exercise, dietary changes, and mind-body techniques such as meditation and yoga. While complementary therapies are not intended to replace medical treatment, they may help to manage symptoms of dementia and improve overall quality of life.

One complementary therapy that has gained attention in recent years is exercise. Research has shown that regular physical activity can improve cognitive function and reduce the risk of developing dementia. Exercise may also improve mood, reduce agitation, and enhance overall physical health in people with dementia.

Dietary changes, such as increasing intake of omega-3 fatty acids and antioxidants, may also be beneficial for managing symptoms of dementia. These nutrients can help to reduce inflammation in the brain and improve cognitive function.

Mind-body techniques, such as meditation and yoga, may also be beneficial for managing symptoms of dementia. These techniques can reduce stress, improve mood, and enhance overall well-being.

It is important to note that while complementary therapies can be beneficial for managing symptoms of dementia, they should not be used in place of medical treatment. It is important to talk with a healthcare provider before starting any complementary therapy, as some may interact with other medications or medical conditions.

In conclusion, alternative and complementary therapies can be useful for managing symptoms of dementia and improving quality of life. While some therapies have shown promise in improving cognitive function, reducing agitation, and enhancing communication, it is important to talk with a healthcare provider before starting any alternative or complementary therapy. Additionally, it is important to note that alternative and complementary therapies should not be used in place of medical treatment, and should be used in conjunction with mainstream medical care.

The role of alternative medicine in dementia care

Alternative medicine, also known as complementary and alternative medicine (CAM), encompasses a range of therapies that fall outside the realm of traditional medicine. People often turn to alternative medicine to manage chronic conditions, including dementia, due to a desire for non-pharmacological options or because traditional treatments have proven ineffective. While alternative medicine approaches to dementia care vary widely, some techniques have shown promise in improving quality of life for people living with the condition.

One alternative medicine technique that has garnered attention in the dementia care community is aromatherapy. Aromatherapy involves using essential oils derived from plants to promote physical and emotional well-being. Studies have found that certain scents, such as lavender and peppermint, can help alleviate anxiety, depression, and sleep disturbances in people with dementia. Aromatherapy can be administered through diffusers, candles, and topical application.

Music therapy is another alternative approach to dementia care that has gained popularity in recent years. Music has been shown to improve mood, reduce agitation and anxiety, and increase social engagement in people with dementia. Music therapy can take many forms, including listening to recorded music, singing, and playing instruments. Some care facilities have even implemented specialized music programs designed for people with dementia, such as the Music and Memory program.

Acupuncture, an ancient Chinese therapy that involves inserting thin needles into specific points on the body, has also been explored as an alternative treatment for dementia. While the evidence is mixed, some studies suggest that acupuncture may help improve cognitive function and reduce behavioral symptoms in people with dementia. Acupuncture is often used in combination with other therapies, such as herbal medicine and massage.

Another alternative medicine technique that has been studied in the context of dementia care is massage therapy. Massage has been shown to reduce stress and anxiety, improve sleep, and increase socialization in people with dementia. Massage therapists can use a variety of techniques, including Swedish massage, reflexology, and aromatherapy, to achieve these benefits.

Herbal medicine, which involves using plants and plant-based extracts to treat illnesses, is another alternative approach to dementia care that has been explored. While there is limited research on the effectiveness of herbal medicine for dementia, some studies suggest that certain herbs, such as ginkgo biloba and sage, may improve cognitive function and reduce behavioral symptoms in people with dementia. However, it is important to note that herbal medicine can interact with traditional medications, so it should only be used under the guidance of a qualified healthcare professional.

In addition to these alternative approaches, there are also a number of complementary therapies that can be used alongside traditional dementia treatments. For example, mindfulness meditation and yoga have been shown to reduce stress and improve mood in people with dementia. Art therapy and reminiscence therapy, which involve engaging with art and past memories, respectively, can also help improve quality of life for people with dementia.

While alternative and complementary therapies can be appealing to people seeking non-pharmacological options for dementia care, it is important to approach these approaches with caution. Many alternative therapies lack scientific evidence to support their effectiveness and can even be harmful if administered incorrectly. It is crucial to consult with a healthcare professional before trying any alternative or complementary therapy, especially if the person with dementia is already taking medication.

In conclusion, alternative and complementary therapies can provide additional options for people with dementia seeking non-pharmacological treatments to improve their quality of life. While some techniques, such as aromatherapy and music therapy, have shown promise in improving mood and reducing behavioral symptoms, it is important to approach these therapies with caution and under the guidance of a healthcare professional. Further research is needed to fully understand the potential benefits and risks of alternative and complementary therapies for dementia care.

Acupuncture, aromatherapy, and other complementary therapies

Acupuncture, aromatherapy, and other complementary therapies have gained popularity in recent years as alternative treatments for various health conditions, including dementia. While there is limited scientific evidence to support their effectiveness, many people with dementia and their caregivers turn to these therapies for relief from symptoms and to enhance overall well-being.

Acupuncture is a traditional Chinese medicine practice that involves inserting fine needles into specific points on the body to stimulate energy flow and promote healing. It has been used to treat a variety of conditions, including pain, anxiety, and depression. Some studies suggest that acupuncture may help with dementia-related symptoms, such as agitation, anxiety, and sleep disturbances. However, more research is needed to determine the effectiveness of acupuncture for dementia and to identify the most appropriate treatment protocols.

Aromatherapy is the use of essential oils extracted from plants to improve physical and emotional well-being. The scents of these oils are believed to have therapeutic effects on the body and mind. Aromatherapy has been used to manage symptoms such as anxiety, depression, and sleep disturbances in people with dementia. Some studies have shown that certain essential oils, such as lavender, can improve sleep quality and reduce agitation in people with dementia. However, more research is needed to establish the efficacy of aromatherapy for dementia and to determine the appropriate dosage and administration methods.

Massage therapy is another complementary therapy that is sometimes used to help manage dementia-related symptoms. Massage can help reduce stress, anxiety, and pain, all of which are common in people with dementia. It can also promote relaxation and improve sleep quality. However, massage therapy should be approached with caution in people with advanced dementia, as they may be more vulnerable to injury or discomfort during massage.

Music therapy is a complementary therapy that involves using music to improve physical, emotional, and cognitive well-being. It has been shown to improve mood, reduce anxiety, and enhance social engagement in people with dementia. Music therapy may also help to stimulate memories and encourage communication. Some studies have shown that music therapy can improve cognitive function in people with dementia, although more research is needed to confirm these findings.

Mind-body therapies, such as yoga and tai chi, are also becoming popular as complementary therapies for dementia. These practices focus on integrating the mind and body to promote relaxation, reduce stress, and improve overall well-being. Some studies have shown that mind-body therapies can improve mood, cognitive function, and quality of life in people with dementia. However, more research is needed to determine the effectiveness of these therapies for dementia and to identify the most appropriate treatment protocols.

While complementary therapies can provide some benefits for people with dementia, it is important to use them in conjunction with traditional medical care and to consult with a healthcare professional before starting any new treatments. Complementary therapies may interact with medications or other treatments and can cause adverse effects if not used appropriately. Additionally, not all complementary therapies are suitable for all people with dementia, and individualized treatment plans are necessary to ensure safety and effectiveness.

In conclusion, acupuncture, aromatherapy, massage therapy, music therapy, and mind-body therapies are among the complementary therapies that are being explored as potential treatments for dementia. While there is limited scientific evidence to support their effectiveness, many people with dementia and their caregivers turn to these therapies for relief from symptoms and to enhance overall well-being. It is important to approach these therapies with caution and to consult with a healthcare professional before starting any new treatments. With further research and development, complementary therapies may become an important part of the treatment and management of dementia in the future.

Evaluating the effectiveness of alternative treatments

Dementia is a debilitating condition that can cause memory loss, confusion, and difficulty with daily tasks. While there is currently no cure for dementia, there are a variety of treatments available that can help manage symptoms and improve quality of life. In recent years, many people have turned to alternative and complementary therapies in search of additional ways to manage dementia symptoms. Below we will we will explore the role of alternative medicine in dementia care, specifically acupuncture, aromatherapy, and other complementary therapies. We will also examine the effectiveness of these treatments and the factors that should be considered when evaluating them.

Acupuncture is a form of traditional Chinese medicine that involves the insertion of thin needles into specific points on the body. Proponents of acupuncture suggest that it can help improve memory, reduce anxiety, and improve overall quality of life for people with dementia. While there is limited scientific evidence to support these claims, some studies have found that acupuncture can be helpful for managing certain symptoms of dementia. For example, a 2016 study published in the Journal of Alzheimer's Disease found that acupuncture was effective in reducing agitation and improving cognitive function in people with Alzheimer's disease.

Aromatherapy is another alternative therapy that has gained popularity in recent years. This practice involves the use of essential oils derived from plants to promote health and well-being. In the context of dementia care, aromatherapy is often used to help reduce anxiety and improve sleep quality. While there is limited scientific evidence to support the use of aromatherapy in dementia care, some studies have suggested that it can be helpful for managing certain symptoms. For example, a 2018 study published in the Journal of Alternative and Complementary Medicine found that aromatherapy was effective in reducing agitation and improving sleep quality in people with dementia.

Other complementary therapies that are sometimes used in dementia care include massage therapy, music therapy, and art therapy. Massage therapy involves the manipulation of soft tissues to improve circulation and promote relaxation. Music therapy involves the use of music to improve mood, reduce anxiety, and promote relaxation. Art therapy involves the use of creative activities to promote self-expression and emotional healing. While there is limited scientific evidence to support the use of these therapies in dementia care, many people find them to be helpful in managing symptoms and improving quality of life.

When evaluating the effectiveness of alternative and complementary therapies for dementia care, it is important to consider a variety of factors. First and foremost, it is important to consult with a healthcare professional before starting any new treatment. This can help ensure that the treatment is safe and appropriate for the individual's specific needs. Additionally, it is important to consider the potential risks and benefits of the treatment, as well as the potential for interaction with other medications or treatments.

It is also important to consider the quality of the scientific evidence supporting the treatment. While some alternative and complementary therapies have been found to be effective in managing certain symptoms of dementia, many of these studies have limitations. For example, some studies may have small sample sizes, making it difficult to draw firm conclusions about the effectiveness of the treatment. Additionally, some studies may not use rigorous research methods, such as randomized controlled trials, which can help to control for other factors that may influence outcomes.

Another factor to consider is the individual's preferences and values. Alternative and complementary therapies can be a helpful addition to dementia care, but they are not suitable for everyone. Some people may prefer more traditional treatments, while others may be more open to trying alternative therapies. It is important to consider the individual's personal preferences and values when deciding on a treatment plan.

In conclusion, alternative and complementary therapies can be a helpful addition to traditional dementia care. Acupuncture, aromatherapy, massage therapy, music therapy, and art therapy are just a few of the alternative therapies that can be used to manage symptoms and improve quality of life

Chapter Twenty-Eight

The Impact of Dementia on Families

Dementia is a complex neurological disorder that affects an individual's cognitive abilities, including memory, language, and decision-making. While the effects of dementia are primarily experienced by the individual with the condition, it also has a profound impact on their family and loved ones. The impact of dementia on families can be emotional, psychological, and financial, and it is important to understand and address these effects to provide optimal care and support.

One of the most significant impacts of dementia on families is the emotional toll it takes. Family members may experience a range of emotions, including sadness, anger, frustration, and grief, as they witness their loved one's cognitive decline. They may also feel a sense of helplessness as they struggle to provide care and support, and may experience feelings of guilt or resentment as their own lives and relationships are affected by the demands of caregiving.

In addition to emotional stress, dementia can also have significant financial implications for families. Caregiving can be costly, with expenses such as medication, medical equipment, and home modifications adding up quickly. Families may also need to hire professional caregivers or make the difficult decision to move their loved one into a long-term care facility, both of which can be expensive.

The impact of dementia on families can also be psychological. Caregivers may experience symptoms of depression and anxiety, and may struggle with social isolation as their caregiving responsibilities limit their ability to engage in other activities. Family members may also experience strain in their relationships, as the demands of caregiving can cause tension and conflict.

Despite the challenges of caring for someone with dementia, many families report feeling a sense of purpose and meaning in their role as caregivers. By providing care and support, family members can help their loved one maintain a sense of dignity and quality of life, and can provide a sense of continuity and stability in the face of a difficult and unpredictable condition.

There are a variety of resources and support networks available to families affected by dementia. Support groups can provide an opportunity for caregivers to connect with others who are going through similar experiences and to share information and advice. Counseling and therapy can help family members manage the emotional and psychological effects of caregiving, and can provide a safe space to express their feelings and concerns.

In addition to support networks, it is also important for families to have access to information and resources about dementia and its management. Education can help families understand the condition and its progression, and can provide guidance on how to provide care and support. Healthcare providers can also play a critical role in providing education and support to families, including information on medications, treatment options, and strategies for managing the symptoms of dementia.

Overall, the impact of dementia on families can be significant and complex, but there are resources and support available to help families navigate this difficult journey. By connecting with support networks, seeking out education and resources, and prioritizing self-care, families can provide the best possible care and support to their loved ones while also taking care of their own emotional, psychological, and financial needs.

Adjusting to a new family dynamic

Adjusting to a new family dynamic is a common experience for families who are caring for a loved one with dementia. Dementia is a progressive condition that affects a person's cognitive abilities, memory, and behavior. As the condition progresses, the person with dementia may require more assistance with activities of daily living, and this can have a significant impact on family members.

One of the challenges that families face is adjusting to a new family dynamic. This can be difficult because the person with dementia may not be able to participate in family activities or may become confused or agitated in social situations. Family members may need to adjust their expectations and routines to accommodate the needs of the person with dementia. This can be challenging, but with support and education, families can learn to adapt to their new circumstances.

It is important for families to seek support from healthcare professionals and dementia support organizations. Healthcare professionals, such as doctors and nurses, can provide guidance on how to manage the symptoms of dementia and offer suggestions on how to adjust to a new family dynamic. Dementia support organizations can provide education, resources, and support to help families cope with the challenges of caring for a loved one with dementia.

One of the most important things that families can do is to communicate openly and honestly with each other. It is important to acknowledge the challenges that everyone is facing and to work together to find solutions.

This can involve making changes to the family's daily routine or seeking additional support from outside sources.

In some cases, families may need to enlist the help of professional caregivers. This can provide much-needed relief for family members who are struggling to manage the demands of caring for a loved one with dementia. Professional caregivers can provide assistance with activities of daily living, such as bathing, dressing, and feeding, and can also provide companionship and emotional support to the person with dementia.

It is important for families to take care of themselves as well. Caring for a loved one with dementia can be emotionally and physically exhausting. Family members should make time for self-care activities, such as exercise, hobbies, or spending time with friends. This can help reduce stress and prevent burnout.

Another important aspect of adjusting to a new family dynamic is managing the financial impact of dementia. Dementia care can be expensive, and families may need to make financial adjustments to accommodate the cost of care. This may involve accessing government benefits or seeking financial assistance from other sources.

In conclusion, adjusting to a new family dynamic when caring for a loved one with dementia can be challenging, but with support and education, families can learn to adapt to their new circumstances. Open communication, seeking support from healthcare professionals and dementia support organizations, enlisting the help of professional caregivers, and practicing self-care can all help families manage the impact of dementia on their family dynamic. It is important to remember that each family's situation is unique, and there is no one-size-fits-all solution. However, with patience, flexibility, and a willingness to seek help when needed, families can successfully navigate the challenges of caring for a loved one with dementia.

Supporting children and young family members

Dementia is a complex and challenging illness not just for the person with the diagnosis, but for their entire family. As such, it is important to provide support not only to the person with dementia but also to their caregivers and loved ones. Children and young family members, in particular, can find the experience of watching their loved one's decline both confusing and distressing. It is essential that they are given appropriate support and guidance to help them understand what is happening and how they can best support their family member.

One of the most important things for children and young family members to understand is that their loved one's behavior and abilities may change as a result of their dementia. This can include forgetting names, getting lost in familiar places, or having difficulty with basic activities of daily living. It can be difficult for children to understand why their loved one is behaving differently, and they may feel frustrated or angry. It is important for caregivers to be patient and compassionate, and to help children understand that their loved one is not behaving this way on purpose.

Another important consideration when supporting children and young family members is to be honest and open about the diagnosis. Depending on the child's age and maturity level, it may be appropriate to explain what dementia is and how it affects the brain. It can be helpful to provide simple, concrete examples of how the person's behavior may change as a result of their dementia, and to emphasize that the person is still the same person they have always been, even if they are behaving differently.

Caregivers can also help children and young family members to understand the importance of maintaining a routine and a sense of normalcy as much as possible. This can include continuing with regular family activities and traditions, even if the person with dementia is no longer able to fully participate. It is also important to encourage children and young family members to continue with their own activities and interests, and to seek out support from other family members, friends, or professional counselors if needed.

Another key consideration when supporting children and young family members is to provide age-appropriate education and resources about dementia. There are many excellent resources available online and in print that can help children understand the illness and learn how to provide support. These resources may include books, videos, or educational websites that are specifically designed for children and young adults.

Finally, caregivers should also be aware of their own needs and the impact of the dementia on their own emotional and physical wellbeing. Caring for a loved one with dementia can be exhausting and emotionally draining, and it is important for caregivers to take care of themselves as well as their loved one. This may include seeking out respite care or other support services, as well as engaging in self-care activities such as exercise, meditation, or spending time with friends and family.

In conclusion, supporting children and young family members when a loved one is diagnosed with dementia is an essential part of providing comprehensive care. It is important to be patient, compassionate, and honest with children, to help them understand the diagnosis and the changes that may occur as a result of the illness. By providing appropriate resources and support, caregivers can help children and young family members navigate this challenging time and build resilience and coping skills for the future.

Strategies for resolving family conflicts

Dementia can have a significant impact on the dynamics of a family. It is a condition that not only affects the individual diagnosed with it but also their loved ones. Family members may struggle with the changes in their loved one's behavior, communication, and cognitive abilities. As a result, family conflicts may arise, adding an additional layer of stress and burden on an already difficult situation. However, there are strategies that families can use to help manage these conflicts and maintain positive relationships.

One of the main strategies for resolving family conflicts in the context of dementia care is open communication. It is essential to have open and honest conversations about the diagnosis, what to expect, and how everyone can work together to provide the best care possible. Family members should share their concerns, fears, and needs, and be willing to listen to each other's perspectives. Misunderstandings can arise when there is a lack of communication, so it is important to keep the lines of communication open.

Another strategy is to involve a third party, such as a social worker or therapist, to help facilitate communication and provide support. These professionals are trained to help families navigate the challenges of dementia care and can offer an objective perspective on the situation. They can help family members understand the diagnosis, the progression of the disease, and the various treatment options available. They can also help families identify and manage any conflicts that may arise.

Setting clear boundaries and expectations can also help to prevent conflicts. Family members should discuss and agree on the roles and responsibilities of each person involved in the care of the individual with dementia. This can include tasks such as medication management, financial management, and caregiving responsibilities. By having a clear understanding of each person's role, there is less room for misunderstandings and conflict.

It is also important for families to take care of themselves. Caregiving can be emotionally and physically exhausting, and it is important for family members to take time for self-care. This can include getting enough sleep, eating well, and engaging in activities that bring joy and relaxation. It is also important for families to seek out support from others, whether that be friends, family, or a support group for caregivers. By taking care of themselves, family members can better manage stress and prevent burnout, which can contribute to conflicts.

In some cases, family conflicts may require the intervention of legal or financial professionals. For example, disagreements over financial management or decisions regarding end-of-life care may require the expertise of an attorney or financial planner. In these cases, it is important for family members to seek out professional help to ensure that the best interests of the individual with dementia are being met.

In conclusion, dementia can have a significant impact on families, and conflicts may arise as a result. However, by using strategies such as open communication, involving third parties, setting clear boundaries, taking care of oneself, and seeking out professional help when necessary, families can work through conflicts and maintain positive relationships. It is important to remember that dementia care is a team effort, and by working together, families can provide the best possible care for their loved one with dementia.

Chapter Twenty-Nine

Dementia and the Media

Dementia is a complex and challenging condition that affects millions of people worldwide. With the increasing prevalence of dementia, the media has an important role to play in shaping public perceptions of the condition and providing accurate information about it. Below we will explore the ways in which the media portrays dementia and its impact on public attitudes towards the condition.

One of the most common ways in which the media depicts dementia is through negative and stigmatizing stereotypes. Dementia is often portrayed as a disease that robs people of their memories, personalities, and independence. This negative portrayal can have a significant impact on people with dementia, their families, and the wider community. It can lead to feelings of fear, shame, and isolation, which can prevent people from seeking help and support.

However, there are also many examples of positive and empowering portrayals of dementia in the media. These stories focus on the strengths and abilities of people with dementia, rather than their deficits. They highlight the importance of providing support and care that allows people with dementia to maintain their dignity, independence, and quality of life.

One of the challenges in media coverage of dementia is the difficulty of accurately portraying the complexity and diversity of the condition. Dementia encompasses a wide range of symptoms and experiences, and affects people in different ways. It can be difficult for the media to capture the nuances and complexities of the condition, and to avoid simplistic or sensationalistic representations.

Another important issue in media coverage of dementia is the need to balance the human interest stories with accurate information and expert analysis. While personal stories can be powerful in raising awareness of dementia and its impact, they can also perpetuate myths and stereotypes if they are not grounded in accurate information and expert insight. It is important for the media to seek out reliable sources and provide accurate and balanced coverage of dementia.

One of the most important ways in which the media can contribute to the fight against dementia is by raising awareness of the condition and promoting research into prevention and treatment. By shining a spotlight on the importance of brain health and the need for more research, the media can help to mobilize public support and drive policy change. It can also help to challenge the stigma and misconceptions that continue to surround dementia.

In recent years, there have been a number of high-profile media campaigns aimed at raising awareness of dementia and promoting research into the condition. These campaigns have included public service announcements, social media campaigns, and media partnerships with organizations working in the field. By using the power of the media to promote positive messages about dementia, these campaigns have helped to change public attitudes and perceptions of the condition.

In conclusion, the media has a vital role to play in shaping public perceptions of dementia and promoting awareness of the condition. While there are challenges and pitfalls in media coverage of dementia, there are also opportunities to promote positive messages and challenge stigma and misconceptions. By working together with experts, advocates, and people with dementia and their families, the media can help to create a more informed, supportive, and understanding society.

Representation of dementia in film and television

Dementia is a complex condition that can be difficult to understand, not only for those living with it but also for their families and caregivers. While it has been the subject of numerous films and television shows, the portrayal of dementia in the media can often be oversimplified or inaccurate. Despite this, media representation can still play an important role in raising awareness about the condition and reducing the stigma associated with it.

One of the most well-known portrayals of dementia in film is the 2004 movie "The Notebook," based on the novel by Nicholas Sparks. The film follows the story of an elderly man, played by James Garner, who reads to his wife, played by Gena Rowlands, from a notebook in an attempt to help her remember their life together. While the movie has been criticized for its unrealistic depiction of dementia, it has also been praised for bringing attention to the emotional toll that the condition can have on families and caregivers.

Another notable film that addresses dementia is the 2014 movie "Still Alice," which stars Julianne Moore as a professor who is diagnosed with early-onset Alzheimer's disease. The film portrays the impact that the diagnosis has on both the individual and their family, and has been praised for its realistic and sensitive portrayal of the condition.

Television has also tackled the topic of dementia, with shows like "The Sopranos" and "Breaking Bad" featuring characters with the condition. However, it is the British television series "Doc Martin" that is often cited as one of the most accurate depictions of dementia on television. In the series, one of the main characters, Aunt Joan, is shown struggling with dementia in a realistic and sensitive way. The show's writers consulted with experts in the field of dementia care to ensure that the portrayal was accurate and respectful.

While these examples provide some insight into how dementia is represented in the media, it is important to note that these are fictionalized accounts and may not accurately reflect the experiences of all individuals living with dementia. Additionally, media representation of dementia can also perpetuate stereotypes and stigma, further adding to the challenges faced by those living with the condition.

Despite these limitations, the media can still be a valuable tool in raising awareness about dementia and reducing stigma. By portraying the emotional toll that the condition can take on individuals and families, these portrayals can help to foster empathy and understanding. In addition, media coverage of new research and breakthroughs in dementia care can help to increase public awareness of the condition and encourage support for further research.

However, it is important to approach media portrayals of dementia with a critical eye, and to seek out accurate information and resources from reputable sources. This can include organizations such as the Alzheimer's Association, which provides information and support for individuals and families affected by dementia, as well as the National Institute on Aging, which funds research on the causes and potential treatments for dementia.

In conclusion, while media representation of dementia can be oversimplified or inaccurate, it can still play an important role in raising awareness about the condition and reducing stigma. By providing a glimpse into the emotional toll that the condition can take on individuals and families, these portrayals can help to foster empathy and understanding. However, it is important to approach media representations of dementia with a critical eye and to seek out accurate information and resources from reputable sources.

The role of media in raising awareness

The media plays a crucial role in raising awareness about dementia, a condition that affects millions of people worldwide. Dementia is a progressive condition that affects a person's memory, thinking, and behavior, and it can have a profound impact on their quality of life. Raising awareness about dementia is essential to improving the lives of people living with the condition, as well as their caregivers and families.

One way that the media can raise awareness about dementia is by providing accurate and up-to-date information about the condition. This can include information about the causes of dementia, the symptoms, and the different types of dementia. It can also include information about the latest research and treatment options, as well as tips for managing the condition.

Another way that the media can raise awareness about dementia is by sharing personal stories of people who are living with the condition. These stories can help to humanize the condition and show the real impact that it can have on people's lives. By sharing these stories, the media can help to reduce the stigma associated with dementia and encourage people to be more understanding and supportive of those living with the condition.

In addition to sharing personal stories, the media can also play a role in advocating for better policies and funding for dementia research and care. By highlighting the challenges faced by people living with dementia and their families, the media can help to raise public awareness and encourage policymakers to take action.

However, it's important for the media to be responsible and sensitive in their coverage of dementia. This includes avoiding sensationalized or stigmatizing language, and ensuring that the information they provide is accurate and evidence-based. It's also important for the media to respect the privacy and dignity of people living with dementia and their families, and to seek their consent before sharing their stories or images.

Overall, the media can play a crucial role in raising awareness about dementia and advocating for better care and support for those living with the condition. By providing accurate and up-to-date information, sharing personal stories, and advocating for better policies and funding, the media can help to reduce the stigma associated with dementia and improve the lives of millions of people around the world.

Influential documentaries and books about dementia

Dementia is a complex and challenging disease that affects millions of people worldwide. While there is no cure for dementia, there are many resources available to help individuals and their families manage the symptoms and challenges that come with this condition. One of the most powerful tools in raising awareness and understanding about dementia is through media, including documentaries and books.

Documentaries can provide a window into the experiences of people with dementia, their families, and the healthcare professionals who care for them. One of the most influential documentaries about dementia is "Alive Inside," which explores the impact of music on individuals with dementia. The film follows social worker Dan Cohen as he brings personalized music to nursing home residents with dementia, showing how music can unlock memories and emotions in even the most advanced stages of the disease. "Alive Inside" has helped to promote the use of music therapy as a non-pharmacological intervention for dementia and has inspired many individuals and organizations to bring music to people with dementia.

Another documentary that has raised awareness about dementia is "His Neighbor Phil," which tells the story of two friends who both have spouses with dementia. The film explores the challenges of caring for a loved one with dementia and the importance of community support in providing care. "His Neighbor Phil" has been praised for its authentic portrayal of the experiences of caregivers and has helped to increase understanding about the impact of dementia on families.

Books are also an important medium for raising awareness about dementia. One of the most influential books about dementia is "The 36-Hour Day" by Nancy L. Mace and Peter V. Rabins. First published in 1981, this book has become a classic resource for families and caregivers of people with dementia. The book provides practical advice for managing the symptoms of dementia and addresses the emotional and psychological challenges of caregiving. "The 36-Hour Day" has helped countless families to navigate the complexities of dementia care and has become a standard reference for healthcare professionals.

Another influential book about dementia is "Still Alice" by Lisa Genova. The novel tells the story of a Harvard professor who is diagnosed with early-onset Alzheimer's disease and explores the impact of the disease on her life and her family. "Still Alice" has been praised for its sensitive portrayal of the experiences of individuals with dementia and their families, and has helped to increase understanding about the challenges of living with the disease.

Documentaries and books about dementia have played an important role in raising awareness and understanding about the disease. By sharing personal stories and experiences, these media have helped to break down stigma and promote empathy and compassion for individuals with dementia and their families. They have also inspired new approaches to dementia care and have provided practical advice and guidance for families and caregivers.

In conclusion, media such as documentaries and books play a significant role in raising awareness and understanding about dementia. They help to bring the experiences of people with dementia and their families to the forefront, promote empathy and compassion, and inspire new approaches to dementia care. As we continue to work towards improving dementia care and finding a cure for this disease, the power of media to educate and inform cannot be underestimated.

Chapter Thirty

Traveling with Dementia

Traveling with Dementia: Challenges and Tips

Traveling is a popular pastime for people of all ages and backgrounds, and this includes those living with dementia. However, traveling with dementia can pose unique challenges that require careful planning and preparation to ensure a safe and enjoyable trip. Below we will we will explore some of the challenges of traveling with dementia and provide tips for making the experience as positive as possible.

Challenges of Traveling with Dementia

One of the biggest challenges of traveling with dementia is the potential for disorientation and confusion. People with dementia may have difficulty navigating new environments, recognizing landmarks or remembering important information, such as the name of their hotel or the location of their belongings. This can lead to feelings of anxiety and fear, which can further exacerbate symptoms of dementia.

Another challenge is the disruption to familiar routines and environments. People with dementia often rely on routine and familiarity to help them feel comfortable and secure. Traveling can disrupt these routines and environments, leading to increased confusion and disorientation.

Finally, traveling with dementia can be physically exhausting. People with dementia may have difficulty adjusting to changes in time zones, sleeping in unfamiliar beds or dealing with long periods of travel. This can lead to fatigue, which can exacerbate symptoms of dementia and make it more difficult to manage.

Tips for Traveling with Dementia

Despite these challenges, there are steps that people with dementia and their caregivers can take to make traveling as enjoyable and safe as possible. Some tips to consider include:

2. Plan Ahead: Plan the trip well in advance and take the time to research the destination thoroughly. This includes researching the local language, customs, and culture, as well as identifying any potential barriers or challenges that might arise.

3. Stick to a Routine: Whenever possible, try to stick to a routine that is similar to the one the person with dementia follows at home. This can include meal times, medication schedules, and bedtime routines. Familiarity can help reduce confusion and disorientation.

4. Pack Wisely: Bring familiar items from home, such as favorite snacks or photos, to help the person with dementia feel more comfortable in new surroundings. Make sure to pack all necessary medications and keep them easily accessible throughout the trip.

5. Consider Special Accommodations: Many travel companies and airlines offer special accommodations for people with disabilities or special needs, including those with dementia. These can include priority boarding, wheelchair assistance, and special seating arrangements.

6. Use Technology: There are many apps and devices available that can help people with dementia navigate unfamiliar environments. GPS trackers, memory aids, and translation apps can all be useful tools when traveling.

7. Take Breaks: Traveling can be physically and mentally exhausting, so it's important to take frequent breaks and allow time for rest and relaxation. This can include scheduling downtime during the day or taking frequent breaks during long periods of travel.

8. Stay Flexible: Travel plans can change unexpectedly, so it's important to stay flexible and be prepared to adjust plans as needed. This can include changing the itinerary to accommodate the person with dementia's needs or being prepared to change accommodations if necessary.

Traveling with dementia can pose unique challenges, but with careful planning and preparation, it can also be an enjoyable and rewarding experience. By sticking to routines, packing wisely, using technology, and staying flexible, people with dementia and their caregivers can help ensure a safe and positive trip.

Preparing for travel with a person with dementia

Traveling with a person who has dementia can be challenging, but it is possible with careful planning and preparation. Travel can be a positive experience for people with dementia, as it can provide stimulation, new experiences, and opportunities for socialization. However, traveling can also be disorienting and overwhelming for people with dementia, and can lead to increased confusion and anxiety. Below we will we will explore some strategies for preparing for travel with a person with dementia.

The first step in preparing for travel with a person with dementia is to consult with a healthcare provider to ensure that the person is healthy enough to travel. The healthcare provider may also be able to provide advice on managing the person's medications, as well as tips for preventing and managing common problems that can arise during travel, such as dehydration, jet lag, and motion sickness.

Another important step is to plan the trip carefully, taking into account the person's individual needs and preferences. This may involve selecting a destination that is familiar or that has familiar activities, or choosing a mode of transportation that is less stressful, such as driving rather than flying. It may also involve selecting accommodations that are comfortable and accessible, and that offer amenities such as familiar food and activities.

It is also important to plan for potential emergencies or unexpected events. This may involve carrying important documents such as medical records and contact information for healthcare providers, as well as packing essential items such as medications, snacks, and water. It may also involve arranging for travel insurance, which can help cover the cost of emergency medical care or transportation.

When traveling with a person with dementia, it is important to be patient and understanding, and to allow for plenty of rest and relaxation. It may also be helpful to involve the person in the planning process as much as possible, and to provide clear and simple instructions throughout the trip.

In addition to these practical strategies, there are also a number of resources available to help people with dementia and their caregivers prepare for travel. For example, the Alzheimer's Association offers a number of travel tips on their website, including advice on preparing for air travel, managing medications, and coping with jet lag. The National Institute on Aging also offers a comprehensive guide to traveling with someone who has dementia, which includes practical advice and helpful resources.

In conclusion, traveling with a person with dementia can be challenging, but with careful planning and preparation, it can also be a positive and rewarding experience. By consulting with healthcare providers, planning the trip carefully, preparing for emergencies, and being patient and understanding, caregivers can help ensure a safe and enjoyable travel experience for everyone involved.

Tips for successful trips and vacations

Traveling with a person who has dementia can be challenging, but it is possible with proper planning and preparation. It is important to remember that people with dementia can still enjoy traveling and experiencing new things, but it requires some extra attention and care to ensure that the trip is safe and enjoyable for everyone involved.

Here are some tips for successful trips and vacations with a person who has dementia:

1. Plan ahead: Before traveling, it is important to do your research and plan ahead as much as possible. Choose destinations that are familiar or similar to the person's routine and interests. Consider the length of the trip, the mode of transportation, and the level of activity involved. Make sure to book accommodations that are safe, comfortable, and accessible.

2. Communicate with the travel company: If you are traveling with a tour group or using a travel company, let them know about the person's condition in advance. This will help them make appropriate accommodations and ensure that the trip is safe and enjoyable for everyone.

3. Pack essentials: Be sure to pack any medications, medical documents, and emergency contact information. Bring familiar items from home such as favorite foods, blankets, and clothing to provide a sense of comfort and familiarity. Bring a list of important phone numbers and addresses, and consider getting a GPS tracker in case the person becomes lost.

4. Schedule breaks: It is important to schedule regular breaks and rest periods throughout the trip. This will give the person with dementia time to rest and recharge, and help prevent overstimulation and fatigue.

5. Involve the person in planning: If possible, involve the person with dementia in the planning process. This will help them feel more in control and engaged, and may help reduce anxiety and confusion during the trip.

6. Be flexible: It is important to be flexible and adaptable during the trip. The person with dementia may experience changes in mood, behavior, or cognition, and it may be necessary to adjust plans or activities accordingly.

7. Be patient and understanding: Traveling with a person who has dementia can be challenging, but it is important to remain patient and understanding. Try to focus on the positive aspects of the trip and enjoy the experience together.

In conclusion, traveling with a person who has dementia requires careful planning, preparation, and flexibility. By following these tips, it is possible to have a successful and enjoyable trip while ensuring the safety and well-being of everyone involved.

Navigating travel challenges and safety concerns

Navigating Travel Challenges and Safety Concerns When Traveling with Dementia

Traveling with a loved one who has dementia can be a daunting task, but it doesn't have to be. With careful planning and preparation, people with dementia can still enjoy traveling and experiencing new things. However, it is important to be aware of the potential challenges and safety concerns that may arise. Below we will we will explore some of these challenges and offer tips for navigating them.

One of the main challenges when traveling with a person with dementia is ensuring their safety. This includes everything from keeping track of their medication and making sure they stay hydrated to preventing wandering and falls. To start, it is essential to speak with the person's doctor before embarking on any travel plans. They can help you develop a plan that takes into account the person's medical condition and any potential risks associated with travel. This might include recommendations for medication management, ensuring adequate hydration, and strategies for preventing falls or wandering.

It is also important to take extra precautions when it comes to transportation. Whether you are traveling by car, plane, or train, it is important to make sure that the person with dementia is seated next to a responsible caregiver who can provide assistance as needed. If you are traveling by car, make sure to plan frequent rest stops and take time to stretch your legs. If you are flying, consider booking non-stop flights and opting for early morning flights to avoid crowds and reduce stress.

Another challenge when traveling with a person with dementia is ensuring their comfort and well-being. This might include finding accommodations that are safe and comfortable for them, as well as ensuring they have access to familiar routines and activities. It is also important to plan ahead for any potential challenges, such as finding wheelchair-accessible transportation or accommodations.

When choosing accommodations, consider the person's needs and preferences. For example, some people with dementia may feel more comfortable in a familiar environment, such as a hotel room that looks similar to their own bedroom. It may also be helpful to choose accommodations that offer amenities like on-site dining, so you can have more control over the person's food choices and schedule.

Finally, it is important to be prepared for unexpected events that may arise while traveling. This might include illness or injury, lost luggage or travel documents, or unexpected changes to travel plans. To prepare for these events, make sure to have a plan in place for contacting emergency services or finding medical care, as well as having copies of important documents like passports and medical records.

In conclusion, traveling with a person with dementia can present unique challenges and safety concerns, but with careful planning and preparation, it is possible to have a successful and enjoyable trip. By working with the person's doctor to develop a travel plan, taking extra precautions when it comes to transportation, choosing accommodations that are safe and comfortable, and being prepared for unexpected events, you can help ensure the person's safety and well-being while on the road.

Chapter Thirty-One

Intimacy and Relationships in Dementia

Dementia is a condition that can cause significant changes in a person's behavior and cognitive abilities, including their ability to communicate and engage in intimate relationships. As a result, intimacy and relationships can become challenging for both the person with dementia and their partner. It's essential to understand the impact of dementia on intimacy and relationships and develop strategies to maintain healthy connections and communication.

Dementia affects a person's ability to remember, think, and communicate. It can also cause changes in mood, behavior, and personality. As a result, people with dementia may struggle to express their emotions and may find it difficult to understand the emotions of others. This difficulty can have a significant impact on their ability to engage in intimate relationships.

For people with dementia who are in long-term relationships, maintaining an intimate connection can be challenging. As the disease progresses, the person's ability to communicate and engage in physical contact may decline. This decline can lead to feelings of isolation and loneliness, both for the person with dementia and their partner.

It's important to note that intimacy can take many forms and is not limited to physical contact. For people with dementia, emotional intimacy, such as sharing memories and experiences, can be just as important as physical intimacy. It's essential to explore different ways of maintaining intimacy that are appropriate and comfortable for both partners.

Caregivers also play a crucial role in supporting intimacy and relationships for people with dementia. Caregivers should be aware of the challenges that dementia can pose to intimacy and relationships and work to provide support and guidance. They can help facilitate communication between partners, provide opportunities for emotional and physical intimacy, and help the person with dementia maintain their sense of identity and self-worth.

It's also essential to acknowledge that intimacy and relationships in dementia care can raise ethical and moral concerns. For example, there may be concerns about the capacity of a person with dementia to provide informed consent to sexual activity or other intimate interactions. Caregivers and healthcare providers should be prepared to address these concerns and work to ensure that all interactions are safe, consensual, and respectful of the person with dementia's dignity and autonomy.

Overall, maintaining intimacy and relationships for people with dementia requires understanding the challenges and developing strategies to address them. Communication, emotional connection, and physical contact are all essential components of a healthy relationship, and it's essential to explore different ways of maintaining these connections as the disease progresses. Caregivers and healthcare providers play a crucial role in supporting intimacy and relationships and should be prepared to address ethical concerns that may arise.

Maintaining intimacy and affection in relationships

Maintaining intimacy and affection in relationships can be a challenge for couples when one partner has dementia. However, it is important to remember that intimacy and affection are essential to human relationships, and can play a key role in the well-being of both partners.

One of the first steps to maintaining intimacy and affection is to acknowledge the changes that may occur as a result of dementia. This can include changes in communication, behavior, and physical ability. It is important to approach these changes with understanding and patience, and to communicate openly about any concerns or feelings.

Communication is a key factor in maintaining intimacy and affection. This can include verbal and nonverbal communication, such as gestures, touch, and facial expressions. It is important to find ways to communicate that work for both partners, and to be patient and understanding when communication becomes more difficult.

It is also important to continue engaging in activities and hobbies that both partners enjoy. This can include going for walks, listening to music, or playing games. These activities can help to maintain a sense of connection and shared experiences.

In addition to communication and shared activities, physical touch can also play an important role in maintaining intimacy and affection. This can include holding hands, hugging, or even just sitting close to one another. Touch can help to provide a sense of comfort and connection, and can also help to reduce stress and anxiety.

As dementia progresses, it is important to adjust expectations and find new ways to maintain intimacy and affection. This may include finding ways to express love and affection through nonverbal cues, such as a smile or a hug. It may also involve finding new activities that are more suited to the changing abilities of the person with dementia.

Maintaining intimacy and affection can be a challenge, but it is essential to the well-being of both partners. With understanding, patience, and communication, it is possible to maintain a deep and meaningful connection, even in the face of dementia.

Navigating changes in sexual behavior and desire

Dementia is a neurological disorder that can have a significant impact on a person's cognitive and behavioral abilities. One aspect of the disease that can be difficult for both patients and their partners is the changes that can occur in sexual behavior and desire. Below we will we will explore the challenges of navigating these changes and some strategies for coping with them.

Dementia can affect a person's sexual behavior and desire in a variety of ways. Some people may experience a decrease in sexual desire, while others may become more sexually aggressive or engage in inappropriate sexual behavior. The disease can also impact a person's ability to communicate their desires or understand the signals of their partner.

For caregivers and partners, these changes can be challenging to navigate. It's essential to recognize that a person's sexual behavior and desire are a normal part of their human experience and should be respected and valued. However, it's also crucial to balance this respect with a need for safety and appropriate behavior.

One strategy for maintaining intimacy and affection in relationships affected by dementia is to focus on non-sexual forms of affection, such as hugging, holding hands, and cuddling. These actions can help provide a sense of physical connection while minimizing the risk of inappropriate behavior.

It's also important to maintain open communication and recognize that a person's needs and desires may change over time. Regularly checking in and asking how a person is feeling and what they need can help build trust and intimacy in a relationship.

Another challenge that can arise is navigating changes in sexual behavior and desire that may be inappropriate or dangerous. In these situations, it's essential to establish clear boundaries and communicate them to the person with dementia. This can be a difficult conversation to have, but it's crucial for the safety and well-being of both parties.

It's important to note that some changes in sexual behavior may be the result of medication side effects or other underlying medical conditions. It's essential to work with a healthcare provider to rule out any underlying medical causes and adjust medications as needed.

Finally, it's essential to recognize that dementia can be a isolating disease that can impact a person's social connections and relationships. Supporting a person's social engagement and maintaining a sense of community can help provide a sense of purpose and connection that can be beneficial for both their emotional and sexual well-being.

In conclusion, navigating changes in sexual behavior and desire in relationships affected by dementia can be challenging, but it's essential to recognize that these changes are a normal part of the human experience. Maintaining open communication, focusing on non-sexual forms of affection, and establishing clear boundaries can help maintain intimacy and affection while ensuring safety and appropriate behavior. Working with healthcare providers to address any underlying medical conditions is also crucial. Finally, supporting a person's social engagement can help provide a sense of purpose and connection that can be beneficial for both their emotional and sexual well-being.

The impact of dementia on spousal and partner relationships

Dementia is a chronic condition that affects a person's cognitive abilities and can lead to significant changes in their personality, behavior, and relationships. When a person with dementia is in a spousal or partner relationship, the impact of the condition on their relationship can be profound. Below we will we will discuss the impact of dementia on spousal and partner relationships and explore strategies for coping with the changes.

The Impact of Dementia on Spousal and Partner Relationships

Dementia can have a significant impact on spousal and partner relationships. One of the most significant changes is the loss of shared memories and experiences. Dementia can cause a person to forget important moments in their lives, including the memories they share with their partner. As a result, the person with dementia may not recognize their spouse or partner, and they may feel like they are living with a stranger.

Another challenge that arises in spousal and partner relationships is the impact of changes in behavior and personality. Dementia can cause a person to become more agitated, aggressive, or paranoid, which can put a strain on the relationship. The partner or spouse may feel that they no longer know how to communicate with their loved one, or they may feel overwhelmed by the changes.

Dementia can also have a significant impact on intimacy and sexual relationships. The person with dementia may lose interest in sex or experience changes in sexual behavior, which can be distressing for their partner. The partner may also feel guilty for having sexual desires when their loved one is experiencing such significant changes.

Strategies for Coping with Changes in Spousal and Partner Relationships

Coping with the changes caused by dementia in spousal and partner relationships can be challenging. However, there are strategies that can help partners and spouses maintain their relationship and cope with the changes.

The first strategy is to seek support. Spouses and partners should consider joining support groups or seeking counseling to help them cope with the changes. Support groups can provide a safe space to talk about the challenges they are facing and provide them with advice and guidance from others who have experienced similar situations.

Another strategy is to focus on the present. When a person with dementia is struggling with memory loss, it can be helpful to focus on the present moment rather than dwelling on the past. Partners and spouses can find new ways to connect and make new memories together, such as going for walks, listening to music, or engaging in other activities that they enjoy.

It is also important to be patient and understanding. Partners and spouses should understand that their loved one's behavior and personality changes are not intentional and are a result of their condition. By being patient and understanding, partners and spouses can avoid becoming frustrated or angry with their loved one.

Finally, it is essential to maintain intimacy and affection in the relationship. Partners and spouses can find new ways to show affection and maintain intimacy, such as holding hands, cuddling, or giving each other massages. By maintaining physical contact, partners and spouses can continue to feel connected and supported.

Dementia can have a significant impact on spousal and partner relationships, causing changes in behavior, personality, and intimacy. However, by seeking support, focusing on the present, being patient and understanding, and maintaining intimacy and affection, partners and spouses can cope with these changes and maintain their relationship. It is important to remember that while the changes caused by dementia can be challenging, they do not have to define the relationship. By adapting to the changes and finding new ways to connect, partners and spouses can continue to support each other and enjoy their relationship.

Chapter Thirty-Two

Dementia and Pets

Dementia is a condition that can be incredibly isolating for those who experience it. It can be challenging to communicate, form new memories, and engage in social activities. However, pets can provide a source of comfort, companionship, and even purpose to people living with dementia.

Pets, especially dogs and cats, have been shown to reduce stress, anxiety, and depression. Studies have shown that petting a dog can lower blood pressure, and even the simple act of watching fish in an aquarium can be calming. Pets can also serve as a source of motivation for people with dementia. Having a pet to care for can provide a sense of purpose and routine.

Pets can also provide a sense of familiarity and comfort. People with dementia may struggle with recognizing family members or their surroundings, but they are more likely to remember their pet's name, and the routine associated with caring for them.

Incorporating pets into dementia care can have a range of benefits, including improved physical health, enhanced emotional well-being, and improved cognitive function. However, it is essential to take appropriate safety measures to ensure both the person with dementia and the pet are safe and happy.

For example, it is essential to select a pet that is a good fit for the person's temperament and living situation. A highly energetic dog might not be a good fit for someone with limited mobility, and a cat might not be suitable for someone with allergies.

It is also essential to ensure that the pet's needs are being met. Dogs need to be walked and fed regularly, and cats need to be groomed and provided with a litter box. If the person with dementia is unable to meet these needs, it may be necessary to hire a pet sitter or consider other options, such as a robotic pet.

Finally, it is crucial to keep safety in mind when introducing pets into dementia care. For example, a person with dementia may forget that they have already fed their pet, leading to overfeeding. Pets may also become agitated or stressed if they are not used to the person's behavior or movements.

Overall, incorporating pets into dementia care can be a powerful tool for improving the well-being of both the person with dementia and their caregiver. However, it is important to take appropriate safety measures and ensure that the pet is a good fit for the person's needs and living situation. With proper planning and care, pets can provide a source of comfort, companionship, and purpose to people living with dementia.

The therapeutic benefits of pets for individuals with dementia

The use of pets as therapy for individuals with dementia has gained popularity in recent years. Studies have shown that pets can provide emotional and psychological benefits to individuals with dementia, leading to improved quality of life. Below we will we will explore the therapeutic benefits of pets for individuals with dementia.

Pets, particularly dogs and cats, have been shown to provide companionship and emotional support to individuals with dementia. They can act as a source of comfort, reduce stress and anxiety, and provide a sense of purpose and meaning to individuals with dementia. Studies have shown that pet therapy can improve mood, reduce behavioral symptoms, and increase social interaction among individuals with dementia.

One study conducted by the University of California, Los Angeles, found that individuals with dementia who received pet therapy had improved cognitive function, including increased memory and attention span. Another study published in the Journal of Psychiatric Research found that pet therapy reduced agitation and improved socialization among individuals with dementia living in long-term care facilities.

Pets can also provide a sense of routine and structure for individuals with dementia. Pets require daily care, including feeding, grooming, and exercise. These tasks can provide a sense of purpose and routine for individuals with dementia, helping them to maintain cognitive and physical function.

Pet therapy can also benefit family members and caregivers of individuals with dementia. Caregiving can be a stressful and emotionally challenging role, and the presence of a pet can provide a source of comfort and support for both the individual with dementia and their caregiver. In addition, pets can facilitate social interaction and provide a sense of normalcy in what can be a difficult and isolating experience.

While pets can provide therapeutic benefits for individuals with dementia, it is important to consider the practical and safety implications of pet ownership. Pets require daily care and attention, including feeding, grooming, and exercise. Individuals with dementia may not be able to provide adequate care for a pet, and may need assistance from family members or caregivers. In addition, pets can pose safety risks, particularly if an individual with dementia is prone to wandering or has a history of aggression.

It is important to carefully consider the individual needs and abilities of the person with dementia when considering pet therapy. Some individuals may benefit from the companionship of a pet, while others may find the responsibility of pet ownership overwhelming. It is also important to consider the temperament and behavior of the pet, as well as any potential health risks, before introducing a pet to an individual with dementia.

In conclusion, pet therapy can provide significant emotional and psychological benefits for individuals with dementia. Pets can provide companionship, reduce stress and anxiety, and improve cognitive function and social interaction. However, it is important to carefully consider the practical and safety implications of pet ownership, and to assess the individual needs and abilities of the person with dementia before introducing a pet. With proper consideration and care, pet therapy can be a valuable and effective tool for improving quality of life for individuals with dementia.

Tips for managing pet care and safety

Tips for Managing Pet Care and Safety in Dementia

Pets are often considered family members and can bring tremendous joy and comfort to people, particularly those living with dementia. Studies have shown that spending time with pets can help reduce stress, anxiety, and depression, improve mood and socialization, and increase physical activity. However, pets also require care and attention, and their presence can pose potential safety risks for people with dementia. Here are some tips for managing pet care and safety in dementia.

Assess the individual's ability to care for a pet

Before introducing a pet into the home, it's important to assess the person's ability to care for a pet. People with dementia may struggle with cognitive and physical abilities necessary for pet care. They may forget to feed or walk the pet, leave doors or windows open, or mishandle the pet. If the person is unable to care for a pet, alternative options such as pet therapy or visits from a trained service animal may be a better choice.

Choose the right pet

Selecting the right pet is crucial for managing pet care and safety in dementia. The pet's breed, size, temperament, and activity level should match the person's ability and lifestyle. For example, a large, high-energy dog may not be suitable for someone who is physically frail, while a quiet, low-maintenance cat may be a better fit.

Ensure proper pet care

Proper pet care is essential for the health and well-being of the pet and the person with dementia. This includes regular feeding, exercise, grooming, and veterinary checkups. It's important to establish a routine for pet care and involve the person with dementia as much as possible. This can help promote a sense of purpose and responsibility, as well as provide opportunities for meaningful interactions with the pet.

Address safety concerns

Pets can pose safety risks for people with dementia, particularly if the person has a tendency to wander or become disoriented. It's important to ensure that the pet is properly secured and that doors and windows are locked. It's also a good idea to have identification tags on the pet and to keep a recent photo of the pet in case it becomes lost.

Provide socialization opportunities

Pets can be a great source of socialization for people with dementia. They can provide opportunities for meaningful interactions with family, friends, and other caregivers, as well as opportunities for community involvement, such as visiting a local dog park or participating in a pet therapy program.

Seek support from a healthcare professional

Managing pet care and safety can be challenging for caregivers, particularly if they are also caring for someone with dementia. It's important to seek support from a healthcare professional, such as a geriatrician or dementia care specialist, who can provide guidance and resources for managing pet care and safety.

In conclusion, pets can provide numerous benefits for people with dementia, including reducing stress, improving mood, and promoting physical activity. However, it's important to ensure that pets are selected and cared for properly and that safety concerns are addressed. With proper management and support, pets can be an important part of a person's life and a valuable source of comfort and companionship.

Animal-assisted therapy and dementia

Animal-assisted therapy has become increasingly popular in recent years as a complementary treatment option for individuals with various health conditions, including dementia. This type of therapy involves using animals, such as dogs, cats, or even horses, as a tool to enhance the physical, emotional, and social well-being of people with dementia. Below we will we will explore the benefits and challenges of animal-assisted therapy for individuals with dementia, as well as the various forms of animal-assisted therapy that are currently available.

One of the primary benefits of animal-assisted therapy for individuals with dementia is that it can help to reduce anxiety and depression. Research has shown that spending time with animals can increase levels of the hormone oxytocin, which can lead to feelings of relaxation and calmness. This is especially important for people with dementia, who may experience high levels of anxiety and depression due to the cognitive and physical changes that come with the disease. Additionally, animal-assisted therapy can provide a sense of companionship and purpose, which can be particularly helpful for people with dementia who may feel isolated and lonely.

Another benefit of animal-assisted therapy is that it can improve socialization and communication skills. Animals are non-judgmental and can help to create a safe and accepting environment for individuals with dementia. This can lead to increased confidence and engagement in social activities, as well as improved communication with caregivers and family members. In addition, animal-assisted therapy can stimulate reminiscence and cognitive function, as interacting with animals can trigger memories and improve mental agility.

While animal-assisted therapy can be incredibly beneficial for individuals with dementia, it is important to note that it also comes with some challenges. One of the primary challenges is ensuring the safety of both the individual with dementia and the animal. This requires careful screening and training of animals, as well as close supervision during therapy sessions. Additionally, it is important to consider the individual preferences and comfort levels of each person with dementia, as not everyone may enjoy or benefit from animal-assisted therapy.

There are several different types of animal-assisted therapy that are currently available for individuals with dementia. One popular form is animal-assisted activities, which involve brief interactions with animals in a supervised setting. This can include petting or playing with dogs, cats, or other animals, and can be a source of relaxation and enjoyment for individuals with dementia. Another form of animal-assisted therapy is animal-assisted education, which involves using animals as a tool for learning and cognitive stimulation. For example, individuals with dementia may be asked to identify different types of animals or recall facts about animal behavior.

Finally, animal-assisted therapy can also take the form of animal-assisted interventions, which are more structured and goal-oriented. This type of therapy may involve training dogs to perform specific tasks, such as alerting their owner to potential safety hazards or providing physical assistance. Animal-assisted interventions may also include group therapy sessions, where individuals with dementia work together with trained animals to achieve specific therapeutic goals.

In conclusion, animal-assisted therapy is a promising and effective complementary treatment option for individuals with dementia. It has been shown to reduce anxiety and depression, improve socialization and communication skills, stimulate cognitive function, and provide a sense of companionship and purpose. However, it is important to carefully consider the safety and individual preferences of each person with dementia when implementing animal-assisted therapy, and to choose the appropriate form of therapy based on their needs and goals. With careful planning and supervision, animal-assisted therapy can be a valuable tool in enhancing the well-being of individuals with dementia.

Chapter Thirty-Three

Dementia and Aging in Place

Dementia is a progressive disease that affects memory, thinking, and behavior. The disease can make it challenging for individuals to perform everyday tasks and make decisions, eventually leading to the need for assistance with daily living activities. Aging in place refers to the ability of an individual to remain in their own home and community as they age, rather than moving into a care facility. For individuals with dementia, aging in place can be a feasible option with proper planning and support.

Living with dementia presents unique challenges, especially for those who want to age in place. While dementia is a progressive disease, many individuals with dementia can live independently with the right support and accommodations. Here are some considerations to help individuals with dementia age in place:

1. Home modifications: Modifying the home to meet the needs of someone with dementia is essential to ensure their safety and independence. Some simple home modifications include installing handrails and grab bars, removing tripping hazards, labeling cabinets and drawers, and adding motion-activated lighting. A dementia-friendly home design can help the individual with dementia navigate their living space easily.

2. Communication: Communication is vital for someone with dementia. Their cognitive abilities may change over time, making it harder for them to communicate effectively. It is essential to use clear, concise language, avoid complicated sentences, and maintain a calm tone when communi-

cating with someone with dementia. Individuals with dementia may also benefit from non-verbal cues, such as visual aids, to help them understand and remember important information.

3. Caregiver support: Providing adequate support to caregivers is crucial when it comes to aging in place with dementia. Caregivers should have access to resources, such as support groups and respite care, to help them manage their loved one's care and maintain their own mental and physical well-being. With proper caregiver support, individuals with dementia can receive the care they need to remain in their homes and communities.

4. Technology: Technology has become increasingly prevalent in dementia care. From smart home devices to GPS tracking systems, technology can help individuals with dementia maintain their independence while aging in place. Smart home devices, such as voice-activated assistants, can help individuals with dementia manage their daily routines and provide reminders. GPS tracking systems can also be helpful in case the individual with dementia wanders off.

5. Social support: Social support is essential for individuals with dementia to maintain their mental health and well-being. Maintaining social connections with friends, family, and community can help individuals with dementia feel connected and engaged. Support from community organizations, such as senior centers and faith-based organizations, can also help provide social support and promote overall well-being.

In conclusion, aging in place with dementia is possible with proper planning and support. Home modifications, effective communication, caregiver support, technology, and social support are essential considerations when supporting individuals with dementia who want to remain in their homes and communities. With the right support, individuals with dementia can maintain their independence and live a fulfilling life as they age in place.

Home modifications for safety and independence

Home modifications for safety and independence are crucial for individuals with dementia who want to age in place. Aging in place refers to the ability of older adults to live independently in their own homes as they age. Dementia can make it challenging to live at home safely and independently, and it is essential to make the necessary home modifications to reduce the risk of accidents and falls.

Some common home modifications that can enhance safety and independence for individuals with dementia include:

1. Lighting: Adequate lighting is essential to prevent accidents and falls. Replace dim lights with bright, energy-efficient bulbs and install night lights in hallways, stairways, and bathrooms.

2. Flooring: Replace slippery floors with non-slip flooring, such as carpet or rubber. Remove area rugs or secure them with non-slip backing.

3. Handrails: Install handrails on both sides of staircases, hallways, and bathrooms to help individuals with dementia maintain their balance.

4. Grab bars: Install grab bars in the shower, bathtub, and near the toilet to prevent slips and falls.

5. Door locks: Replace traditional locks with easy-to-use locks or keyless entry systems to prevent individuals with dementia from getting locked in or out of their homes.

6. Kitchen modifications: Install cabinet locks and childproof latches on cabinets and drawers to prevent access to hazardous items like knives and cleaning supplies. Also, install a sensor to detect when the stove is left on.

7. Bathroom modifications: Install a raised toilet seat to make it easier for individuals with dementia to sit and stand. Use a shower chair or bench in the shower or bathtub.

8. Technology: Use technology to enhance safety, such as smart home technology that can detect falls or alert caregivers if an individual with dementia wanders.

These home modifications can help individuals with dementia maintain their independence and reduce the risk of accidents and falls. However, it is essential to work with a qualified occupational therapist or home safety specialist to determine the appropriate modifications for each person's unique needs.

In addition to these physical modifications, it is also essential to consider the social and emotional aspects of aging in place for individuals with dementia. This can include providing social support, engaging in meaningful activities, and ensuring that basic needs like nutrition and healthcare are met.

One way to provide social support is through the use of respite care, where a caregiver can take a break while a substitute caregiver provides care for the individual with dementia. This can provide the caregiver with time to recharge while also ensuring that the individual with dementia receives the care they need.

Engaging in meaningful activities can help individuals with dementia maintain their cognitive and social abilities. This can include hobbies, exercise programs, or social events specifically designed for individuals with dementia.

Finally, ensuring that basic needs like nutrition and healthcare are met is essential for individuals with dementia who want to age in place. This can include working with a healthcare provider to manage any medical conditions or medications, as well as providing nutritious meals and ensuring that the home is clean and safe.

In conclusion, home modifications for safety and independence are crucial for individuals with dementia who want to age in place. Physical modifications like lighting, flooring, and handrails can enhance safety, while social and emotional support can help individuals with dementia maintain their cognitive and social abilities. It is essential to work with a qualified occupational therapist or home safety specialist to determine the appropriate modifications for each person's unique needs. With the right modifications and support, individuals with dementia can maintain their independence and quality of life as they age in place.

In-home care services and support

As dementia progresses, it can become challenging for individuals to perform daily activities and manage their healthcare needs. This is where in-home care services and support can play a crucial role. In-home care refers to a range of services provided to individuals who require assistance with activities of daily living, such as bathing, dressing, and medication management. Below we will we will discuss the different types of in-home care services available for individuals with dementia and their families.

One of the most common types of in-home care is personal care services. Personal care services can include help with bathing, dressing, grooming, toileting, and feeding. These services are provided by a home health aide or personal care assistant. Home health aides are trained professionals who can provide basic medical services such as taking vital signs and administering medication. Personal care assistants are not medically trained, but they can provide support with non-medical tasks such as housekeeping, meal preparation, and running errands.

Another type of in-home care is skilled nursing care. Skilled nursing care is provided by licensed nurses who can provide medical services such as wound care, medication management, and intravenous therapy. Skilled nursing care can be especially important for individuals with dementia who may have complex medical needs.

In addition to personal care services and skilled nursing care, there are also respite care services available for caregivers. Respite care services provide temporary relief for family members or caregivers who need a break from caregiving responsibilities. Respite care can be provided in the home or in a residential care facility, and can range from a few hours to several days.

Another important aspect of in-home care for individuals with dementia is specialized dementia care. Specialized dementia care can include services such as memory care, specialized therapy, and support groups. Memory care services provide a safe and supportive environment for individuals with dementia, while specialized therapy can help improve cognitive and physical abilities. Support groups can also provide emotional support for individuals with dementia and their families.

When considering in-home care services, it is important to consider the needs and preferences of the individual with dementia as well as their family. Some individuals with dementia may prefer to receive care from a familiar caregiver, such as a family member or friend. Others may prefer the professional care of a home health aide or personal care assistant. It is also important to consider the level of care needed and the cost of services.

There are also different types of in-home care agencies to consider. For example, some agencies provide services on an hourly basis, while others provide 24-hour care. Some agencies specialize in a particular type of care, such as dementia care or hospice care. It is important to research different agencies and their services to find the best fit for the individual with dementia and their family.

In addition to in-home care services, there are also other types of support available for individuals with dementia and their families. For example, many communities offer adult day care services, which provide a safe and stimulating environment for individuals with dementia while their caregivers are at work or taking a break. There are also respite care facilities available that can provide temporary care for individuals with dementia.

In-home care services can play a crucial role in supporting individuals with dementia and their families. These services can help individuals with dementia maintain their independence and quality of life, while also providing support and relief for their caregivers. It is important for families to consider the different types of in-home care services available and to work with healthcare professionals to develop a care plan that meets the unique needs of the individual with dementia.

Strategies for successful aging in place

As people age, they often face a range of challenges that can affect their ability to live independently, and those with dementia may face even more difficulties. However, aging in place - remaining in one's own home as opposed to moving into a care facility - can offer numerous benefits for people with dementia, including increased comfort, familiarity, and a sense of control over their surroundings. With the right strategies and support, aging in place can be a successful and fulfilling option for many individuals with dementia.

One of the key components of aging in place for those with dementia is ensuring that the home environment is safe and supportive. This may involve making modifications to the home, such as installing handrails or grab bars in the bathroom, removing tripping hazards, and providing adequate lighting. It can also involve purchasing assistive technology, such as medical alert systems or automatic medication dispensers, that can help the individual with dementia maintain their independence and stay safe.

In addition to modifying the home environment, in-home care services can also be a crucial component of successful aging in place for individuals with dementia. Caregivers who are specially trained in dementia care can provide assistance with activities of daily living, such as bathing and dressing, as well as offer companionship and engage the individual with dementia in meaningful activities. Home health aides can also monitor the individual's health and wellbeing, and alert family members or healthcare providers if any concerns arise.

Another important aspect of successful aging in place for those with dementia is providing opportunities for socialization and engagement. This may involve scheduling regular visits with family and friends, participating in community activities or programs, or engaging in hobbies and interests that the individual with dementia enjoys. It can also involve utilizing resources such as adult day care centers, which offer structured socialization and activities for individuals with dementia while also providing respite for caregivers.

Providing support for family caregivers is also essential for successful aging in place for individuals with dementia. Family caregivers often experience significant stress and burnout, and may need assistance with tasks such as managing medications, coordinating care, and navigating the healthcare system. Providing respite care - temporary relief from caregiving duties

- can also be beneficial for both the caregiver and the individual with dementia.

Finally, it is important to recognize that aging in place may not be a viable option for everyone with dementia, particularly as the disease progresses. As such, it is important for individuals and families to have a plan in place for the eventual transition to a care facility if necessary. This can involve researching and visiting potential facilities, working with healthcare providers to identify the right level of care, and making financial and legal preparations for the move.

In conclusion, aging in place can be a successful and fulfilling option for individuals with dementia with the right strategies and support. Ensuring a safe and supportive home environment, utilizing in-home care services and resources, providing opportunities for socialization and engagement, and supporting family caregivers are all crucial components of successful aging in place. However, it is important to recognize that aging in place may not be an option for everyone, and planning for the eventual transition to a care facility is an important part of the process.

Chapter Thirty-Four

Supportive Living Environments

Supportive living environments can be a vital resource for individuals with dementia who may require specialized care and assistance with daily activities. These environments aim to provide a safe and comfortable home-like setting for individuals with dementia, while also offering the necessary resources and support to help them live as independently as possible.

One type of supportive living environment is a memory care community. Memory care communities are specifically designed to cater to the needs of individuals with dementia, offering specialized care and activities that are tailored to their unique requirements. These communities typically provide a range of services, including 24-hour monitoring, assistance with daily activities such as dressing and bathing, medication management, and social and recreational activities that are designed to promote cognitive stimulation and engagement.

Assisted living communities are another type of supportive living environment that can be beneficial for individuals with dementia. These communities offer a range of services that can be tailored to the needs of individuals with varying degrees of independence, from those who require minimal assistance to those who require round-the-clock care. In addition to providing assistance with daily activities, assisted living communities typically offer social and recreational activities, as well as access to on-site medical care and other support services.

In addition to memory care and assisted living communities, there are also supportive living environments that cater specifically to individuals with dementia who also have other medical conditions or disabilities. For example, some supportive living environments may be designed for individuals who require assistance with mobility or who have medical conditions that require specialized care, such as diabetes or heart disease.

Regardless of the type of supportive living environment, these communities can be an excellent resource for individuals with dementia who require additional support and assistance. By offering a safe and comfortable living environment that is designed to meet their unique needs, supportive living environments can help individuals with dementia to maintain a sense of independence and quality of life, while also providing the necessary resources and support to help them manage their condition.

It is important to note, however, that supportive living environments can be expensive, and not all individuals with dementia may have access to these types of resources. In some cases, government-funded programs or community-based organizations may be able to provide support and assistance to individuals with dementia who require specialized care but are unable to afford it.

In addition to supportive living environments, there are also a variety of other resources and services that can be beneficial for individuals with dementia and their caregivers. These may include respite care, which can provide temporary relief to caregivers who may require a break from their caregiving responsibilities, as well as community-based programs and support groups that offer education, resources, and emotional support to individuals with dementia and their families.

Types of long-term care options for individuals with dementia

Dementia is a progressive disease that affects the brain and causes memory loss, communication difficulties, and impaired judgment. As the disease progresses, individuals with dementia may require long-term care to meet their needs. There are several options available for long-term care, and families and caregivers must consider each option carefully to ensure that the individual with dementia receives the best care possible.

One of the most popular long-term care options for individuals with dementia is assisted living facilities. These facilities are designed for individuals who require assistance with daily living tasks, such as bathing, dressing, and medication management. They also provide meals, housekeeping, and social activities. Assisted living facilities can be a good option for individuals with dementia who are still relatively independent but require some assistance.

Nursing homes are another long-term care option for individuals with dementia. These facilities provide more advanced medical care and around-the-clock nursing care. Nursing homes are ideal for individuals who require a higher level of care, such as those with advanced stages of dementia. Nursing homes provide specialized care for individuals with dementia, including medication management and behavioral interventions.

Memory care units are specialized units within assisted living or nursing home facilities that provide care for individuals with dementia. These units are designed to meet the unique needs of individuals with dementia, including a secure environment, specialized care, and programming that focuses on memory care. Memory care units provide a safe and supportive environment for individuals with dementia and can help slow the progression of the disease.

In-home care is another option for individuals with dementia who wish to age in place. In-home care providers offer a range of services, including personal care, medication management, and companionship. In-home care allows individuals with dementia to remain in their homes and receive the care they need while maintaining a sense of independence.

Adult day care programs are also available for individuals with dementia. These programs provide care and social activities during the day while allowing individuals to return home in the evenings. Adult day care programs can be a good option for individuals who require supervision during the day but can manage at home with the help of family or friends.

Respite care is a short-term care option that provides temporary relief for caregivers. Respite care allows caregivers to take a break from their caregiving responsibilities while ensuring that their loved one receives the care they need. Respite care can be provided in an assisted living facility, nursing home, or in-home care setting.

When considering long-term care options for individuals with dementia, families and caregivers must consider the individual's needs, preferences, and the level of care required. They should also consider the cost of care, the location of care, and the availability of specialized dementia care services.

Evaluating and selecting a care facility

As dementia progresses, individuals with the condition may require more support and care than their loved ones can provide. This can lead to the difficult decision of whether to move the person with dementia to a care facility. Choosing the right care facility for a loved one with dementia is a critical decision that requires careful evaluation and consideration. Below we will we will discuss the process of evaluating and selecting a care facility for individuals with dementia.

The first step in evaluating care facilities for individuals with dementia is to gather information about different facilities in the area. One way to do this is to use online resources, such as the Medicare Nursing Home Compare website. This website provides information on the quality of care and services provided by different nursing homes and skilled nursing facilities. It is important to review the ratings and read reviews from other families who have used these facilities.

Another important step is to visit the facility in person. It is recommended to schedule a tour with the facility and ask questions about the care and services provided. Some important questions to ask include:

What is the staff to resident ratio?

What type of training do the staff members receive to work with individuals with dementia?

What activities and programs are available for residents?

What is the policy on family involvement in care and decision-making?

During the visit, it is important to observe the interactions between staff and residents. Look for signs of compassion, respect, and attentiveness. Also, take note of the cleanliness and organization of the facility.

It is also important to consider the specific needs of the individual with dementia. Some facilities specialize in caring for individuals with dementia and offer specialized programs and services. Other facilities may not be equipped to provide the level of care needed for individuals with advanced dementia. Consider the individual's level of functioning, behavior, and medical needs when evaluating care facilities.

Another important factor to consider is the cost of care. Care facilities can be expensive, and it is important to understand the costs and payment options before making a decision. Some facilities accept Medicare and Medicaid, while others require private payment. Be sure to ask about any additional fees or costs that may not be included in the basic rate.

Once you have gathered all of the necessary information, it is time to make a decision. It is important to involve the individual with dementia and their family in the decision-making process. The individual with dementia may have specific preferences and needs that should be considered. Family members can provide valuable insights into the individual's history and personality, which can help in selecting the right facility.

It is also important to have a plan for transitioning to the care facility. This can be a difficult and emotional process for both the individual with dementia and their family members. It is important to communicate with the staff and develop a plan for gradually transitioning the individual to the facility. This may include spending time at the facility before the move or bringing familiar items from home to make the new environment feel more comfortable.

Transitioning to a new living environment

Transitioning to a new living environment can be a challenging experience for anyone, but it can be particularly difficult for individuals with dementia. Dementia is a progressive brain disorder that affects memory, thinking, behavior, and daily functioning. As the disease progresses, individuals with dementia often require more assistance with daily activities and may need to move to a new living environment that can better meet their care needs. Below we will we will explore the challenges associated with transitioning to a new living environment for individuals with dementia, as well as strategies for making the transition as smooth as possible.

The challenges of transitioning to a new living environment for individuals with dementia can be significant. Moving to a new environment can be confusing and disorienting for individuals with dementia, who rely on familiarity and routine to help them navigate their daily lives. The new environment can be overwhelming and stressful, leading to anxiety, depression, and behavioral changes. Family members and caregivers may also experience emotional distress as they help their loved one navigate the transition.

To help make the transition to a new living environment as smooth as possible, there are several strategies that families and caregivers can use. The first step is to involve the individual with dementia in the decision-making process as much as possible. This can help the person feel more in control of the situation and may reduce anxiety and stress. It is important to provide information and support throughout the decision-making process and to allow the person to express their preferences and concerns.

Once a decision has been made, it is important to prepare the individual with dementia for the move. This can include providing information about the new environment, showing pictures or videos of the new home, and arranging for visits to the new location. It may also be helpful to have familiar items from the old home, such as photographs or favorite objects, in the new environment to provide a sense of familiarity and comfort.

Another important strategy is to maintain a consistent routine as much as possible. This can help individuals with dementia feel more comfortable and secure in their new environment. Familiar activities and routines can also help reduce confusion and anxiety.

It is also important to provide emotional support and reassurance throughout the transition. Caregivers can help individuals with dementia by offering encouragement and support, listening to their concerns, and acknowledging their feelings. It may also be helpful to involve a social worker or other professional to provide additional support and guidance.

In addition to these strategies, there are also resources available to help families and caregivers navigate the transition to a new living environment. Local support groups and community organizations can provide information and support to help individuals with dementia and their families during the transition. Healthcare providers, such as doctors and social workers, can also provide guidance and resources to help families and caregivers make informed decisions.

Chapter Thirty-Five

Staying Informed and Up-to-Date

Staying informed and up-to-date is crucial when it comes to understanding and managing dementia. As new research, therapies, and treatments emerge, it is important for patients, caregivers, and healthcare professionals to stay informed in order to make the best decisions for those affected by dementia. Below we will we will explore various ways to stay informed and up-to-date in regards to dementia.

One of the most important ways to stay informed about dementia is to stay connected with healthcare professionals. Regular check-ups and appointments with doctors, nurses, and specialists can provide valuable information on the progression of the disease and any new treatments or therapies that may be available. Additionally, healthcare professionals can provide advice on how to manage symptoms and behaviors associated with dementia, as well as offer support and resources for caregivers.

Another way to stay informed is to attend seminars, conferences, and workshops. Many organizations, including the Alzheimer's Association and the Lewy Body Dementia Association, host events that offer the latest information on research, treatments, and care practices. These events also provide an opportunity for caregivers and patients to connect with others who are going through similar experiences.

Online resources are also a valuable tool for staying informed about dementia. The internet offers a wealth of information on the latest research, treatments, and care practices. Many reputable organizations, such as the National Institute on Aging and the Mayo Clinic, offer information on their websites about dementia and related conditions. Caregiver forums and support groups are also available online, providing an opportunity for individuals to connect with others and share their experiences.

Social media can also be a useful tool for staying informed about dementia. Many organizations, including the Alzheimer's Society and the Alzheimer's Association, have active social media accounts where they share the latest news and research about the disease. Additionally, social media can be a useful platform for connecting with others who are going through similar experiences and sharing information and resources.

Books and documentaries are another way to stay informed about dementia. Many authors and filmmakers have shared their personal experiences with dementia, offering valuable insights into the disease and its impact on individuals and families. These resources can provide an emotional connection and a deeper understanding of the challenges and successes that come with caring for someone with dementia.

Finally, staying informed about dementia also means staying informed about policy and advocacy efforts. Organizations such as the Alzheimer's Association and the National Institute on Aging advocate for research funding and policy changes that can improve the lives of those affected by dementia. By staying informed about these efforts, individuals can get involved and help drive change.

Keeping current with dementia research and news

Dementia is a progressive brain disorder that affects millions of people worldwide. As researchers continue to learn more about this condition, there is a growing body of information and news about advances in diagnosis, treatment, and prevention. Keeping up with the latest research and news can be important for individuals living with dementia, their families and caregivers, and healthcare professionals.

One way to stay informed about dementia research and news is to regularly check reputable sources such as government agencies, academic institutions, and non-profit organizations. These sources often publish updates on new research findings, clinical trials, and treatment options. For example, the National Institute on Aging (NIA) and Alzheimer's Association are both excellent resources for reliable and up-to-date information on dementia.

Another way to stay informed is to read news articles and features on dementia. These articles can provide insights into the latest developments in research, as well as personal stories about individuals living with dementia and their caregivers. However, it is important to be discerning when reading news articles, as not all sources are reputable or accurate.

Social media can also be a valuable tool for staying informed about dementia. Many organizations, researchers, and individuals share news, updates, and personal stories on platforms like Twitter and Facebook. Following reputable sources and engaging in conversations with other individuals in the dementia community can help to stay up-to-date on new developments and best practices.

Attending conferences and events focused on dementia can also provide an opportunity to learn about the latest research and connect with others in the field. Conferences such as the Alzheimer's Association International Conference (AAIC) and the International Dementia Conference bring together researchers, healthcare professionals, and individuals living with dementia to share their insights and experiences.

It is important to note that the field of dementia research and care is constantly evolving, and not all news and research findings will be relevant or helpful for every individual living with dementia. It is important to approach new information with a critical eye and consult with healthcare professionals before making any changes to treatment plans or care routines.

In addition to staying informed about the latest research and news, it is also important to be aware of local and national resources and services available for individuals living with dementia and their families. Many non-profit organizations and government agencies offer support groups, educational programs, and other services to help individuals living with dementia and their caregivers navigate the challenges of the condition.

Some organizations also offer newsletters or email updates that provide information about local events and resources. For example, the Alzheimer's Association offers an e-newsletter that provides updates on research and news, as well as information about local support groups and events.

The role of conferences, seminars, and workshops

The field of dementia research and care is constantly evolving, with new information and techniques being developed all the time. Professionals and caregivers alike must stay informed in order to provide the best possible care for those living with dementia. One valuable way to stay up-to-date is through attending conferences, seminars, and workshops.

Conferences and seminars are typically larger events that offer attendees the opportunity to learn about new research and innovations in the field of dementia care. These events often feature presentations from leading experts, as well as opportunities for networking and collaboration with other professionals. Seminars may be more focused on specific topics, such as a particular type of dementia or a specific aspect of care. They may also be shorter in duration than conferences.

Workshops, on the other hand, are often more hands-on and practical. They may involve training in specific skills or techniques, such as communication strategies or activities for people with dementia. Workshops may be led by experienced professionals, such as occupational therapists or dementia care specialists, and can be a valuable way for caregivers to learn new skills and techniques.

Attending these events can be beneficial for both professionals and caregivers. Professionals can gain new insights and knowledge about the latest research and techniques, which they can then apply to their work with patients. They can also connect with other professionals in the field, which can lead to new collaborations and partnerships.

Caregivers, on the other hand, can learn new skills and techniques to better care for their loved ones with dementia. They can also connect with other caregivers who are going through similar experiences, which can be a valuable source of support and encouragement.

There are a variety of conferences, seminars, and workshops available for those interested in learning more about dementia care. Some are geared towards professionals, while others are open to anyone interested in the topic. Many organizations that focus on dementia research and care offer these types of events, including the Alzheimer's Association and the Lewy Body Dementia Association.

In addition to in-person events, there are also a variety of online resources available for those interested in staying up-to-date on the latest research and techniques in dementia care. Webinars and online courses can be a convenient way to learn from leading experts without having to travel to a physical location. Online support groups and forums can also be a valuable way for caregivers to connect with others and share experiences and advice.

It's important to note that attending conferences, seminars, and workshops can come with a cost, both in terms of registration fees and travel expenses. However, many organizations offer scholarships and other forms of financial assistance to help offset these costs. Caregivers may also be able to find local events that are more affordable and accessible.

In addition to attending events, there are a variety of other ways to stay informed about dementia research and care. Reading scientific journals and other publications can be a valuable way to stay up-to-date on the latest research. Following organizations and experts on social media can also be a convenient way to receive regular updates and news.

Tips for staying informed and connected within the dementia community

Dementia can be a complex and challenging condition to manage, and staying informed and connected within the dementia community is essential for caregivers, families, and those living with dementia. As new research emerges and treatment approaches evolve, it is critical to stay up-to-date on the latest developments to provide the best possible care and support.

One of the most effective ways to stay informed about dementia is to become involved in community-based organizations that focus on dementia education, support, and research. These organizations provide a wealth of information on the latest research findings, treatment options, and support services available to those affected by dementia. They also offer opportunities to connect with others in similar situations, share experiences, and learn from others who have navigated similar challenges.

Another way to stay informed is by attending conferences, seminars, and workshops focused on dementia. These events bring together experts in the field of dementia research and care to share the latest research and best practices for managing the condition. Attending these events provides an opportunity to learn from leading experts, network with other caregivers and professionals, and gain new insights into the latest advances in dementia care.

Additionally, there are many online resources available for those seeking information about dementia. Online communities, support groups, and forums offer a space for caregivers, families, and those living with dementia to connect and share their experiences. These online resources can provide a wealth of information on the latest research findings, new treatment options, and practical tips for managing the condition.

It is essential to be mindful of the sources of information when seeking information about dementia. Reliable sources of information include national and international organizations that specialize in dementia care, research, and support. These organizations typically provide accurate, up-to-date information that has been vetted by experts in the field. However, it is essential to be cautious when seeking information from non-accredited sources, such as blogs or social media. Always verify the accuracy of the information and seek advice from a medical professional before making any decisions about treatment or care.

Finally, it is important to recognize the importance of self-care and support when navigating the challenges of dementia. Caring for a loved one with dementia can be emotionally and physically demanding, and it is crucial to seek support and take care of one's mental and physical health. Taking time to engage in activities that bring joy and relaxation, seeking support from friends and family, and connecting with other caregivers can help prevent burnout and maintain overall well-being.

In conclusion, staying informed and connected within the dementia community is essential for caregivers, families, and those living with dementia. Community-based organizations, conferences, seminars, and workshops, online resources, and reliable sources of information can provide a wealth of information on the latest research, treatment options, and support services available to those affected by dementia. Additionally, self-care and support are critical when navigating the challenges of dementia care. By staying informed and connected, caregivers and families can provide the best possible care and support to their loved ones living with dementia.

SD - #0033 - 121026 - C0 - 229/152/17 - PB - 9781776969265 - Matt Lamination